Why

Can't I

Stop

EATING?

Why
Can't I
Stop
EATING?

Recognizing, Understanding, and
Overcoming Food Addiction

Debbie Danowski and Pedro Lazaro, M.D.

HAZELDEN

Hazelden
Center City, Minnesota 55012-0176

1-800-328-0094
1-651-213-4590 (Fax)
www.hazelden.org

Library of Congress Cataloging-in-Publication Data
Danowski, Debbie, 1965–
    Why can't I stop eating? : recognizing, understanding, and
    overcoming food addiction/Debbie Danowski and Pedro
    Lazaro.
        p. cm.
    Includes bibliographical references and index.
    ISBN 13: 978-1-56838-365-1
    1. Compulsive eating. 2. Twelve-step programs. I. Lazaro,
Pedro, 1956– II. Title.

RC552.C65 D36 2000
616.85'26—dc21
                                                    99-086746

Editor's note
All the stories in this book are based on actual experiences.
The names and details have been changed to protect the privacy of the people involved. In some cases, composites have
been created.

10 09 08 07   11 10 9

Cover design by Terri Kinne
Interior design by Donna Burch
Typesetting by Stanton Publication Services, Inc.

*This book is dedicated to everyone who suffers
from the disease of food addiction
and to those who tease them.
May they all find their way.*

Contents

Acknowledgments

A book like this is not the effort of any one person. There have been many people along the way who have helped and supported me in my work. I'd like to thank some of them specifically: I wouldn't have been able to survive both the writing and marketing process if it were not for the unwavering encouragement and enthusiasm of my husband, Fred Danowski. His willingness to read and critique my work before anyone else, and at all hours of the night, made writing this book easier. And his honesty, even when I didn't want to hear it, helped me to grow both as a person and as a writer. Equally crucial is his complete faith in me and my work. No words can describe how much his support has meant to me throughout our nearly nine years together.

The love and support (yes, I mean financial too!) of my parents, Ann and Andy, were also critical in the development of this book. Their unconditional help, even when they were sure I should be committed for the choices I had made, was and continues to be the guiding force of my writing career.

Similarly, the comments and encouragement from my sister, Karen, and brother-in-law, Danny, helped to make even my darkest moments bearable. They helped me to believe when everything seemed impossible. Along with them, my niece, Melissa, has taught me so many valuable lessons about taking time to play and have fun. Our trips to carnivals and amusement parks have been an extremely important and enjoyable part of my recovery process.

My brother, Mike, and his wife, Denise, who supported me through difficult times and gave me hope and encouragement were another important part of this process. So many other members, both living and deceased, of my family also made this book possible with their belief in and encouragement of me.

My friends have also provided an enormous amount of support. Some of these include Kellie and Shawn Sharnick who listened to me when I needed to talk; Bev Robillard who read everything I've written since high school; Liz Biles who typed pages in the initial book proposal; Dawn Rosner and Pat Myer for their skillful editing; Jennie Hendrix, Lisa Wolk, Rich Mayo, Sally Michlin, Paulette Day, Chris O'Hearn, and Mark Egmon for their undying encouragement exactly when I needed it most; Fred and Marie Danowski for their help during difficult times; my group of friends from Mondays, Wednesdays, and Fridays who gave me the unconditional love I needed to live; Charles Kurmay for making sense of legal issues; and Mike Greene for helping me understand the physiological aspects of food addiction.

Professionally, this book would not be what it is today without the initial guidance of Stacy Prince. Her patience and suggestions improved the quality of my writing tenfold. Likewise, encouragement from my coauthor, Dr. Pedro Lazaro, was an important part of the publishing process. The willingness of Deborah Coffin to support my work was also invaluable during the initial stages. And the honesty of those mentioned in chapter 8 provided valuable insight into the disease of food addiction. Though many chose to remain anonymous or use pseudonyms, I know exactly who they are and their help has saved at least one food addict from death—me.

This book would never have made it to press without the belief and support of several very important people at Hazelden. First, Jerry Spicer's willingness to forward the manuscript to Darlene Gish, who developed a strong belief in the material, provided the groundwork for this book. It was Corrine Casanova's support, dedication, and skillful editing that polished this manuscript, but it was her strength and commitment that allowed this to evolve into a published book. And Catherine Broberg's skillful copyediting added the needed finishing touches.

I would also like to express my undying gratitude to everyone who was a part of my initial recovery, but most especially to Linda P., Phil W., Martha O., Linda B., and Marge P. I met them as an angry, fat, hopeless child, but with their love, support, and guidance, I found hope and enthusiasm and became ready to face a life I didn't know was possible: free from the chains of food addiction. Similarly, I am grateful for Pat Demeyan and Dolores Smith for their help in guiding me through life in recovery.

I would like to thank several people at Sacred Heart University for giving me the opportunity to teach what I love. Dr. David Curtis, Dr. Marian Calabrese, Dr. Louise Spence, Dr. Sylvia Watts, and Dr. Jacqueline Rinaldi have provided valuable guidance, support, and understanding throughout my time at the university. There is one person at Sacred Heart without whom I could never have written my first publishable word: Dr. Ralph Corrigan, who believed in my writing from the first minute I walked into his freelance writing class, has consistently served as not only a great source of strength but a role model as well.

And finally, there are no words to express my gratitude to God for the life and work He has given me.

—Debbie Danowski

Introduction

"Why can't I stop eating?" It was a question I had asked myself each day for the last twenty-three years as I struggled desperately to lose weight. No matter what I did, it didn't seem to help. Overwhelming physical cravings dominated my life. I was powerless to stop eating, and I hated myself for it.

At 328 pounds, I rarely looked in the mirror below my neck for fear of seeing the massive rolls of fat that made up my enormous body. No matter how tight my clothes got or how severely my body ached, I continued to eat massive amounts of food.

In public, I constantly had a smile plastered on my face to hide the humiliation I felt. In private, my life was a constant cycle of bingeing. Filled with self-hatred, I had contemplated suicide many times. If I had to continue living like this, I no longer wanted to go on.

As my final effort, I decided to try a new program I had heard about. If this didn't work, I planned to eat myself to death. There was no other answer for me. I was sure I would die fat and alone. . . .

It has been more than ten years since I felt like that. After discovering the program I mentioned, my life changed completely. It is no longer dominated by food cravings, and I live a happy, productive life I never dreamed possible. Today, my life is truly a miracle.

While taking a pill to lose weight or going on a crash diet may seem like the answer to all of our prayers, in reality, it's not. There is a completely natural alternative to dangerous diet drugs and starvation plans. And unlike expensive weight-loss plans, this program is available without high fees or dangerous side effects.

What, you haven't heard? While much media attention is given to diet drugs and fad weight-loss plans, little, if any, has been written about the craving-free alternative. What? You don't know? No one's told you that you can obtain the same benefits without a two-dollar-a-day pill habit or expensive packaged food? You don't know that it isn't necessary to endanger your health in order to lose weight?

Well, take heart. There is hope! You don't have to risk your life in order to be thin. It is possible, as you have read on the previous page, to live a life completely free of food cravings without taking any pills or starving yourself. You won't have to spend hundreds, or even thousands, of dollars to lose weight, and you will not be asked to purchase specially packaged food.

Your life will be your own. You won't be driven to eat everything in sight anymore. Your head will be clear and you'll have hope. Life will no longer be about eating as much food as you can stuff in your mouth before someone notices. And you will never again be chained to the refrigerator night after night, desperately searching for that one perfect food that will make you feel whole.

And if that's not enough, you will also be free of the dangerous side effects that come with introducing diet pills into your system or starving yourself. You will not be plagued with memory loss. Your heart will not race uncontrollably, and depression will not overwhelm you. Your mouth will not constantly be dry, and diarrhea will not frequently affect you. But most important of all, you will not be putting your life in danger.

With our program, you will not be exposed to any of these

dangers. Instead, you will be shown a completely natural way to obtain the benefits of weight loss and sane living. You will learn that it is possible to lose weight and keep it off without using pills. What could be better?

So, what do you have to do? What is required of you to achieve all of these benefits? Well, for right now, it's very simple. Just continue reading! In the first several chapters, you will be shown the medical evidence behind our program.

Then, after you have all of the facts, you will discover the natural alternative to the diet methods you have been using— a program that will free your body from its physical need for certain types of food. For all of this, you're only asked to keep reading! Can you handle that?

Why

Can't I

Stop

EATING?

1

First, the Facts

What causes your physical cravings for food? Why can't you seem to control them? To answer these questions, it's vital that you understand what happens in your body when you eat certain foods. The next two chapters will present an overview of your physiological system and how it causes you to physically crave food. Then, the third chapter will examine the medical research and theory behind the cravings. Read on and discover why you can't stop eating!

One of the most important facts we have learned about food over the years is that certain foods react negatively in a person's system, which causes the person to overeat. As soon as these substances enter the system, a person physically craves more and more of them, and no matter how much is eaten, it will never be enough. Just as an alcoholic physically craves alcohol, some people physically crave certain foods. (For our purposes throughout the book, we will address these people as "food addicts.")

It is this physical craving for substances that causes individuals to overeat. In the same manner that, after years of drinking, alcoholics become dependent on alcohol, food addicts desire food. This establishes the phenomenon of "craving" described by Dr. William D. Silkworth in "The Doctor's Opinion" section of *Alcoholics Anonymous*. Silkworth notes that alcoholics drink "to overcome a craving beyond their mental control."[1]

Those who have struggled for years to lose weight can relate this description to food. How many times have you told yourself that you weren't going to overeat only to find yourself doing just that within a matter of minutes?

There are things that happen within all of our bodies that we cannot control. When we cut ourselves, we bleed. Each night we all need a certain amount of sleep or we will become exhausted the next day. Some of us experience hormonal irregularities once a month during menstruation, while others suffer from allergies, diabetes, chronic bronchitis, cancer, or heart disease. All of these are things we cannot control, though we may take preventive measures.

Some are simply biological facts, while others are inherited illnesses, about which we have no choice. Your food problem is exactly the same. You have no choice about the physiological makeup of your body. You did not ask to be sensitive to certain foods, and until now, you did not know about these sensitivities. In other words, *it is not your fault that you are fat,* but it is your responsibility.

To put it bluntly, the time has come for you to stop blaming yourself for something you cannot change and to begin changing something you can. After you have read the facts about food sensitivities, the responsibility to act is completely yours, but the blame is not.

Physiologically Addictive Foods

Physical food cravings were recognized in the medical community as far back as 1985, when Drs. David B. Herzog and Paul M. Copeland published an article in *The New England Journal of Medicine* noting differences in the brain chemical makeup of some individuals.[2] They cited several studies involving animals which proved that manipulating brain chemicals reduced the animals' appetite for certain foods.

What does this have to do with you? It means that some people are physiologically predisposed to overeat. In other words, the chemical makeup of your body may cause you to eat certain foods in abundance. While your mind may be telling you not to eat that cupcake, your body, because of its needs, is overpowering your intellect.

Intellectually, you know that eating the cupcake will cause you to gain weight, make you break out, and even make you feel guilty. Biologically, however, you are unable to resist your need to eat. You may even eat a whole dozen, while still knowing all of this. Your physiological needs have caused you to abandon all rational thinking when certain foods are involved.

Sugar

What are these foods? Many studies show that sugar is one of the most physiologically addictive substances.[3] *The New York Times* best-seller *Sugar Busters!* deals with the physical addiction to sugar. Though the medical evidence outlined in this book supports the physical addiction claim, the food plan it describes, for reasons which will be discussed later, is not an effective eating method for those physically addicted to sugar. Once sugar is ingested, the physical craving to eat more and more is so intense that a person with this problem must have larger and larger amounts of sugar as time goes on.

If you are like most food addicts, you are probably telling yourself right now that you do not eat that much sugar. At first, most are sure that since they do not eat candy or other traditional "junk foods" all of the time, they don't have a problem with sugar.

The fact is that nearly every kind of packaged food contains sugar.[4] According to the U.S. Department of Agriculture, the average American consumes more than 151.7 pounds of sugar per year. Additionally, U.S. sugar consumption has been rising at a rate of more than 1.7 percent per year for the last decade while the population growth rate has increased by only about .8 percent. This means, overall, Americans are eating more sugar than ever before. Do you think you are any different?

Perhaps you try to eat low-fat foods, so you think sugar isn't a problem. But in many cases, low-fat foods contain more sugar than "regular" ones to provide enhanced flavor. Sugar is added to foods that you would normally consider to be healthy.

Did you know that canned corn and peas have sugar? Pre-packaged pasta mixes and rice dishes also contain sugar. Taco mixes, ketchup, some crackers, pasta sauces, pickles, ham, tuna mixes, baked beans, frozen breaded fish fillets, specialty coffee mixes, flavored potato chips, tartar sauce, salad dressing, bar-becue sauce, steak sauce, and even some spices may contain sugar.

This is by no means a complete listing. It is only meant to show you how extensively sugar is used in food, to help you see which foods you are eating that contain hidden sugar. Keep in mind that some items listed are available in brands without sugar.

Did you recognize any of the foods listed as those you eat more frequently than others? Are there any that you cannot seem to stop eating? Do you crave several of these foods even after you are full? The reason for this is the addictive nature of sugar. Though the medical profession has yet to reach a con-sensus, there is sufficient evidence to support the addictive biochemical effect sugar has on the body. Sugar is even in-cluded alongside morphine and cocaine in a listing of mind-active drugs written by Dr. Andrew Weil and Winifred Rosen.[5] They define a drug as any substance that in small amounts produces significant changes in the body, mind, or both.

However, they are not the only medical professionals to rec-ognize sugar as an addictive substance. Wholistic and natural food advocates hold very strong beliefs about sugar. One doc-tor, when discussing the reasons some children are more prone to ear infections than others, stated that children are com-monly addicted to sugar and that cravings for the substance can be so overwhelming that children may refuse to eat unless foods with sugar are present.[6] He advised parents to keep their children away from sugar, regardless of their health.

In one Duke University study, it was proved that people who are trying to diet are more likely to overeat sweet foods.[7] Think about the foods you overeat. Most food addicts rarely eat too much cottage cheese or lettuce. As well as causing you to overeat, sugar is also a depressant. It reacts similarly to alcohol in your body. In the same way that you might feel energetic and excited when you first have a few drinks, you also feel "high" after eating sugar. But it is the same empty elation that comes with drinking alcohol. Think back to the last "big" meal you had. How did you feel afterward? Remember your last holiday dinner? What did everyone do after gorging themselves? Sleep? Even those who do not suffer from sugar sensitivities sometimes need to nap after eating large amounts of sugar. The physiological reasons for this will be discussed in the following chapter. For now, just realize that sugar is, for some people, what alcohol is to an alcoholic.

Flour

Other physiologically addictive food substances include white flour, caffeine, wheat, and refined carbohydrates.[8] Because the additives used in processing these foods affect physical aspects of the body, these foods are categorized as mood-altering substances. And their effects are very powerful. According to Dr. Robert Lefever and Marie Shafe, refined carbohydrates and white flour are 20 percent as strong as refined sugars in mood-alteration tendencies.[9]

With statistics like this, is it any wonder that bagels, muffins, and croissants are America's favorite breakfast foods? Think for a minute about what you like to eat for breakfast. Many people on diets start with a bagel every morning. Most addicts believe that one little bagel (especially the small frozen kind) can't hurt them because it doesn't contain a lot of calories. The problem is that many times they cannot stop with one bagel. In some cases, the problem food is disguised "innocently" as low calorie or wheat bread, but flour of any type is still processed and thus contains addictive additives. Additionally, some food addicts may be addicted to wheat, making this a double-edged problem.

These seemingly harmless items that were traditionally believed to be diet foods actually cause a physiological reaction that compels an addict to eat more. Let's talk about one of the most popular flour-filled foods. How often are you able to eat just one piece of pizza? How many times a week do you order pizza with the excuse of it being an easy meal when you really can't wait to taste the luscious treat? And how do you feel after you have "had a few"? Lethargic? Tired? Depressed?

Refined carbohydrates, such as pasta, are another substance that can be physiologically addictive. Experts agree that people who are addicted to sugar are also addicted to refined carbohydrates due to the similar chemical makeup of the two.[10]

Carbohydrate sensitivity is just beginning to be recognized. Prior to this, medical professionals had recommended high-carbohydrate, low-fat diets to combat obesity. For a person addicted to refined carbohydrates, this is a deadly prescription. In a way similar to sugar, when you ingest refined carbohydrates, you set up a cycle of craving. You eat carbohydrates, so you crave carbohydrates, so you eat more carbohydrates, which makes you want even more carbohydrates, so you eat more. . . . Get the picture? The more you eat, the more you crave, the more you eat.

This information makes it clear why some people can't seem to lose weight. Think about how much pasta you eat. Is one small portion ever enough? If not, refined carbohydrates are most likely a problem for you.

Caffeine

Perhaps the most well-known physiologically addictive substance is caffeine. Studies throughout the years have shown that when caffeine use is stopped, withdrawal symptoms occur.[11] And for those of you saying that you do not consume that much caffeine, consider that these symptoms are reported with doses as low as 100 mg per day—the equivalent of one cup of coffee, two cups of tea, or three cans of caffeinated soft drinks.[12]

This brings us to an important point: diet sodas, unless specifically stated, contain caffeine. When first told about caffeine addiction, most food addicts insist that they do not have a problem with it, especially if they hate coffee and never drink tea. Then they discover that the bottles of soda they guzzle endlessly or the chocolates they binge on regularly are loaded with caffeine.

Furthermore, did you know that caffeine is an appetite stimulant? How many late-night binges have you had while drinking soda or coffee? Have you ever drank only black coffee to lose weight? How long did this last?

How many mornings do you drink a cup of coffee to get you going? Or, on those late worknights, do you automatically reach for a soda or cup of tea because you need to be awake? In addition to disrupting your natural biological system, your use of caffeine is setting up a physical dependence that will cause withdrawal symptoms when you stop using it. These symptoms include headaches, mood changes, pain, stiffness, lethargy, and fatigue.

Alcohol

Alcohol is another addictive substance. Dr. Robert Lefever and Marie Shafe describe alcohol as "the ultimate refined carbohydrate." They note that it is unsafe for those with food addictions to drink alcohol.[13] Even if a person never had problems with alcohol, they point out, drinking it may trigger a physiological reaction in the body that will result in overeating.

While some medical professionals say wine is safer than other types of alcohol, the fact remains that for a person addicted to sugar, any type of alcohol is dangerous. Besides the possible physical cravings, alcohol use creates emotional consequences. For instance, as someone who regularly "soothes" himself or herself with food, you may find it easy to replace this emotional crutch with alcohol. In other words, someone who is an addict must always be careful not to exchange one addiction for another, and allowing yourself to have "just one" drink occasionally may, at some point, turn into a full-fledged addiction.

Fats

You have heard the medical research that excessive fat consumption is dangerous and may contribute to heart disease.

We have all been told to decrease our consumption of saturated and unsaturated fats. But what does this mean? What is the nutritional difference between the two kinds of fat, and which is better?

The answer may surprise you, considering all the media attention fats receive. According to Dr. Michael A. Schmidt, saturated fats are those that remain solid at room temperature. These are the ones we usually link to heart disease. Unsaturated fats are those that are liquid at room temperature and found in vegetable oils.[14] Schmidt points out that our bodies can make all the saturated fat and most of the unsaturated fat they need except essential fatty acids, which must be obtained through our diets. Fatty acids are found in such foods as safflower and flax seed oil.

It is the nonessential fatty acids where most of the problems occur. These are the artificially created fats found commonly in doughnuts and pastries. Does Dunkin' Donuts call out your name? If so, you may have a problem with fats.

Giving Up Your Favorite Foods

At this point, you may be feeling slightly overwhelmed with the information presented. It is important to remember that no food is bad, just maybe bad for you. You may even be feeling angry about the prospect of having to give up your favorite foods. Most food addicts are. They hate anyone who tells them that sugar, flour, wheat, and carbohydrates are problems for them. They want to run and hide from this news and most important, they want all of their favorite foods to come with them.

It's important to remember that, if you've tried every other diet in the world and nothing has worked, this could be the answer you have been searching for. Even if you do not want to admit this is possible, think about the types of foods you overeat. Do they all contain sugar, flour, refined carbohydrates, or fats? How many times have you binged on salad unless it was soaked with oil or grated cheese?

In the next chapter, you will learn about the physiological

ways these foods affect your body. For now, the best thing to do is to continue reading. You are probably scared of what you will find, but remember awareness is the key to action, and isn't it time you began taking action?

As you have read, what motivates most food addicts to finally make changes is the amount of pain they experience. What about you? How many times have you eaten something you previously swore to yourself that you would not? Do you try every new diet available only to end up gaining even more weight? Are you depressed over your body size? Do you constantly think about and crave food? Have you put your life on hold until that magical day when you will finally be thin? Do you feel guilty or ashamed about eating in front of others?

The above questions are for you to consider. If you have answered yes to any of them, you probably have a problem with food. If you are a true food addict, you are thinking about food even as you read this. You may even be thinking about your next meal. It is things like this that you need to be aware of, beginning now. Take a few minutes and think about your relationship with food. Think about all of the things you have done to get food and all of the times you have tried dieting. Awareness is the key.

Food Addiction

Before we continue, a few concepts need to be made clearer. In the previous information, we have used the terms "food sensitivity" and "food addiction" interchangeably for ease of reading. The definition of both, in this book's context, is a physical and emotional dependence on food as a way of altering moods to the extent that normal daily functioning is disrupted.

By "normal daily functioning" we mean several things. For example, many addicts avoid going out a lot so they can stay home and eat. Some people are unable to hold a job because they miss work too many times in order to stay home and eat. Others have stolen food to have what they wanted to eat. Lying about the amount of food eaten or pretending to be sick to get more food disrupts normal daily functioning.

And you? Have there been times when you have been "too tired" to attend work or school, only to find yourself home, eating the entire day? Do you wake up late at night to eat when everyone else is asleep? Are your favorite foods hidden throughout the house to make sure no one else eats them? Do you eat small meals in front of others while eating before or after them to make sure you have enough food?

These are only some of the tricks many food addicts use in an attempt to hide their disease. And that is exactly what it is—a sickness. You have no more asked for this sickness than a person who has cancer. Your overeating is a biological malfunctioning of your system, not a character flaw. This is perhaps the hardest and most important message to understand. It helps most addicts to review their relationship with food. For many, the same messages kept coming up: if they could have changed it, they would have. They had tried every diet available, with no success. Instead of looking for the flaws in their diets, all those years of failed attempts have led food addicts to believe that they are morally bankrupt, weak-willed, disgusting people.

Today, we know that is not true. Food addicts are people with a physiological sensitivity to certain foods that react negatively in their system. Willpower has nothing to do with it, and neither does moral character. Again we say, *it is not your fault you are fat*. You can't change your biological makeup, but you can change your tendencies. As a person with cancer must undergo radiation therapy, a food addict must avoid certain substances.

This does not mean you must give up eating delicious meals, but rather that you find substitutes that will not react badly in your system. Why should you? What is in it for you?

A New Life

Imagine a life where food is not the main focus. Imagine that each morning when you wake up, you feel alive and enthusiastic about the day ahead, instead of dreading the bad things you believe may happen. Imagine being able to say no to rich, sweet foods without feeling deprived or angry. But, most of all, imagine living the wonderful, exciting life you were destined to live instead of being trapped by your need to overeat.

Today, as I write this, I have enjoyed more than ten years of complete freedom from constantly thinking about food. Only in a few specific cases, during highly emotional times, have I even emotionally craved any sort of food. I can think clearly and remember more than I ever thought possible.

When I wake up in the morning, I am excited to start the day. I do not dread what will happen. I no longer run to the refrigerator the minute I get out of bed, nor is eating the last thing on my mind before I go to sleep. I do not miss work because of overeating, and I no longer lie, steal, or manipulate to get food. I hold my head up high when I eat in restaurants, and I do not eat before or after I go out for meals. While at first I was afraid to bring my cup and scale into a restaurant, today I know that weighing and measuring my food in a public place is a lot less "degrading" than carrying around an extra 150 pounds.

The food I eat satisfies me. I do not go through the day hungry or wondering how I can eat more. After more than thirty years of life, I finally know what it feels like to be full. I have enough food to eat, and I am satisfied by the taste of it. I enjoy my meals, but I do not obsess over them. I eat three normal-sized meals at the usual times of day, and I do not find it necessary to snack in between. I am active and no longer trapped by my massive size, doing things I had only dreamt of before.

I tell you this not to brag, but to give you hope. If someone had told me ten years ago that I would be thin and free from obsessing about food, I would not have believed them. In my wildest dreams, I never imagined that it was possible to get through even one day without obsessing about food, never mind the past ten years. I did not believe it was possible until I saw it in other people.

For you, I am trying to be that other person. I remember the relief I felt when I found out that other people had done the sick things with food that I had. I experienced joy when I finally knew there was hope.

Now it is your turn. You have heard the evidence, and now you have to decide what to do with it. It is your choice. Do you want to continue to suffer as you have, or are you ready for a change? Would you like to know how your body reacts to those substances mentioned, or do you want to continue to pretend that you do not have a problem? Are you ready to be helped? Do you want to change your life in ways that you can only imagine?

If so, then read on. It's about time you knew these things, but more than that: *You have a right to understand how these substances react in your body.* Ultimately, you will have to make a decision about your relationship with food. For now, the best thing you can do is be willing to read the information in this book. Then, when you have done that, as always, the choice will be yours.

2

The Research

Now that you basically understand how your body reacts to food, it's time to discover the medical research about food addiction. To make an informed decision about your future, you need to know all of the facts, beginning with very early studies about dieting, then, working up to those involving brain chemicals.

While you have probably heard that dieting doesn't work, did you ever wonder where that idea came from? Several medical studies have shown that dieting increases cravings for highly palatable foods, often leading to overeating.[1] In other words, the methods you have been using to lose weight have actually had the exact opposite effect on your body. This fact has been known since World War II, when a physiologist, Ancel Keys, from the University of Minnesota conducted a study.[2]

In his study, Dr. Keys took a group of healthy men and put them on a well-balanced diet, consisting of half of their usual caloric intake. To him, this was classified as "semistarvation," but it is actually quite similar to today's commercial diets.[3] Interestingly enough, when these men were allowed to stop dieting, they massively overate, consuming up to five meals and five thousand calories a day until they returned to their normal weight.[4]

It is important to note that these men were young and healthy and not diagnosed with any food-addiction tendencies. Imagine, then, what the results of this study mean for someone with food sensitivities. How many times have you gained weight when you have gone off a diet? And more important, has your overeating been even worse immediately after dieting?

This happens because your body is unable to distinguish between dieting and life-threatening starvation. When you begin a low-calorie diet, your body goes into starvation mode. Your body's metabolism slows down during this mode. You need fewer calories to maintain the body at rest and fewer calories to produce body heat after eating.[5] When dieting ceases or extra calories are taken in, more of these calories are stored as fat.[6]

In other words, the minute you resume eating more, you will begin gaining weight, which will make dieting even harder next time. It is possible, then, for an overweight person to be gaining weight while eating only 850 calories a day. Additionally, on traditional diets you lose both fat and muscle. Since muscle requires more calories to maintain than fat, muscle loss further decreases both your metabolism and your daily caloric requirements, inadvertently causing a weight gain.[7]

Think for a second about what a lifetime of dieting could do to your body's metabolism. How many diet programs have you tried? If you are like most addicts, you have tried everything from the all-protein diet to the commercially packaged-food one, each time ending up feeling worse than the time before and wondering why the diets never worked.

The intention here is not to slander diets and dieting programs. In some cases, they work for people who are not addicted to food. For a food addict, however, dieting is similar to banging your head against a stone wall—the pain is immense, but the progress is nonexistent. No matter how hard you try, if you are a food addict, traditional dieting will not help you. If you are a food addict, there is no way a conventional diet could have helped you.

Read that last line again and again and again until you really understand it. You were absolutely powerless to stop overeating because of the way certain substances react in your body. Now it is time to discover what happens to you when you eat certain foods.

The "Happy Stuff"

First, we will offer an overview of the physiological process of food addiction in the following example. The technicalities will be left out to make it more understandable. Following that, we will explain the physiological process of food addiction, complete with medical terminology.

Each person's body contains chemicals to make the person feel relaxed, happy, and sleepy. For now, we will call this the "happy stuff." We all need the happy stuff to feel good or relaxed. Some people, for reasons that will be discussed later, do not have enough of these chemicals.

These people feel pain more acutely, are more likely to become depressed, and are, oftentimes, more anxiety prone than those who have enough of the happy stuff. Somewhere along the line, usually at a young age and most times unconsciously, the people lacking the happy stuff find an outside source to obtain it. The results are amazing.

They are finally able to feel relaxed, sleepy, peaceful, and happy. When they have this substance in their bodies, all feels right with the world. And their bodies, once having to struggle to compensate for the decreased amount of the happy stuff, can now relax. They no longer have to send distressing messages to the brain. The happy stuff is there to make everything feel great.

When there is not enough of these chemicals, or the body does not feel like doing the work to make it, a message is sent to the brain to get more of the substance. As time goes on, the body begins to make less and less of its own happy stuff. It depends instead on an outside supply, until finally losing its ability to manufacture it. At this point, the person's life becomes overwhelmed with the constant search for the happy stuff to feel good.

Something has changed inside the person's body. Consuming the happy stuff does not always feel good anymore. In fact, sometimes it feels miserable. The person suffers emotionally from being obsessed with getting the happy stuff. The physical effects of consuming an unnatural amount of the substance are also quite severe. Many times, the person suffers from a loss of memory, obesity, self-induced vomiting, starvation, depression, loss of self-esteem, lack of enthusiasm, decreased energy levels, and low metabolism levels, to name a few. Despite these devastating consequences, the person still continues bringing the happy stuff into his or her body.

Why is this? How can a sane person continue to abuse his or her body in this way? The person's situation is similar to that of the alcoholic who has lost control over drinking. This person's body physically craves the happy stuff, and when he or she does not get it, withdrawal symptoms occur. This person has lost all power to resist the happy stuff. His or her body is unable to make much, if any, of it naturally. Since everyone needs the happy stuff to survive, this person is forced, through physical and emotional cravings, to get it from outside sources. The person becomes a complete slave to it and can no longer control his or her intake of certain substances that make the happy stuff. As with a drug addict, this person's body chemistry is altered in such a way that abstaining from the substance causes the body to revolt. This person is completely powerless over his or her physiological need for the happy stuff.

The amazing thing about all of this is that the person does not even know the name of the happy stuff. Unlike the alcoholic, this person does not realize that it is possible to become addicted to the substance. All this person knows is that his or her body craves certain substances, but not others. There is not anyone to tell this person that he or she is addicted to the happy stuff. No one can easily put a name to the substance, yet the person is routinely criticized for his or her physical appearance.

Instead of receiving the same medical compassion given to an alcoholic or drug addict, this person is branded weak-willed and undisciplined and is constantly mocked in public for something uncontrollable. To deal with this, the person turns to the happy stuff, as he or she always has, to feel better. It no longer works; still the person cannot stop using.

Serotonin

You've probably guessed that the substance we are referring to as "happy stuff" has to do with food. When we eat certain foods, our bodies manufacture the happy stuff, which is actually a brain chemical called serotonin. Serotonin is responsible for regulation of mood, pain, sleep, and appetite.[8]

Let's begin with the basics before we discuss serotonin in depth. There are two parts to your brain. The new brain, called the cortex, is where your thoughts, decisions, and ideas come from. The old brain, the hypothalamus, is where primal instincts such as anger, thirst, fear, sex, and hunger are initiated. In the hypothalamus, and throughout your body, you have neurons—the smallest part of nerve cells. Two parts of a neuron, dendrites and axons, carry electrical impulses to and from the center of the neuron. These impulses send messages to your brain through the gaps, called synapses, that separate the neurons in your body. To carry the messages between the neurons, we have chemicals that travel across the gaps, which are called neurotransmitters. They travel from the ends of nerve fibers to stimulate the following ones. There are receptors to receive the neurotransmitters.

Think of it as a long chain with gaps that is held together by chemicals. The chemical is responsible for getting the message from one nerve to the next. Remember the game called "Telephone"? When one message was passed through several people, it was nearly indistinguishable by the end of the line. Fortunately, our bodies, in most cases, are much more efficient.

In the telephone game, the receivers are an important part of the telephone line. Similarly, in your body, it is the receptors that alter the message. Addiction occurs when these receptors are chemically changed, causing a malfunction with certain neurotransmitters. In chapter 1, you read about a study from *The New England Journal of Medicine* that determined that people with eating disorders have differences in their brain chemical makeup. In food addicts, the neurotransmitter serotonin functions differently than in other people. According to nutrition researchers, serotonin is the brain chemical that calms people down by easing their feelings of stress and tension.[9] Food addicts, as already mentioned, have abnormal serotonin levels, which causes their bodies to seek outside sources of the chemical. Their low serotonin level predisposes food addicts to overeat.[10]

In other words, if you have a serotonin abnormality, you will physically, and probably emotionally, crave large amounts of food, which will lead to a binge. The emotional cravings will be discussed in depth in a later chapter. Up to this point, we have refrained from using the word "binge" until we examined the medical aspects of food addiction. A binge is defined as the unhealthy eating of food. Usually, but not always, it involves consuming large amounts of food at one sitting.

While most of us realize that eating two boxes of cookies is a binge, we may not know that eating six grapefruits is also a binge. It is important to note that binges do not always involve so-called junk food. Eating large amounts of one food at a time is considered nutritionally unhealthy, as a well-balanced diet is needed.

Bingeing on salad, while not outwardly appearing so, is just as serious as bingeing on chocolate. Though the foods do react differently in your system, a binge of any kind carries with it both physical and emotional ramifications. These will be discussed later in this chapter and throughout the book.

Another interesting point is that not all food addicts binge; some do what is known as "grazing" instead. These are the people who will take the entire day to eat a whole cake. Grazers, as the name suggests, eat several smaller meals instead of large amounts of food at one sitting. While someone who binges will eat a lot of food all at once, a grazer will go back to the food several times before it is completely eaten. Though the methods of eating may differ, the physiological results are the same.

Physical Cravings

Let's examine what happens in your body when you eat certain foods. For the sake of brevity in the following discussion, sugar and refined carbohydrates will be referred to simply as carbo-hydrates. Considering that forms of sugar, such as glucose, fructose, and sucrose, are carbohydrates, this seems a logical labeling system.[11]

Non-refined carbohydrates, including natural starches such as soybeans, artichokes, avocados, potatoes, barley, beets, and brown rice are not included in this labeling system. They do not react the same way in your body as refined carbohydrates.

When you eat carbohydrates, your pancreas releases insulin which decreases the concentration of amino acids in your bloodstream—except for tryptophan. This process, in turn, manufactures serotonin.[12]

Since the pancreas is stimulated abnormally, too much in-sulin is released to deal with the excess sugar.[13] Consequently, there is a drop in your blood sugar level due to the removal of the sugar from your bloodstream. This results in feelings of weakness, hunger, headaches, and trembling.[14] Each time this occurs, your cravings for carbohydrates cause you to eat more of the same.[15] Combine that with the increase of serotonin being produced in your system and you have a better idea of a food addict's physiological makeup.

In addition to the cravings, most food addicts report being especially susceptible to physical illnesses. This occurs because carbohydrates, more specifically sugar, are believed to depress your immune system. Think about your own life. Do you get sick more frequently than others?

If you are like I was, you are probably having a lot of doubts about most of the things you have read up to this point. Even though I immediately experienced the actual physical benefits of removing carbohydrates from my body, it was at least three months before I was convinced that I really was addicted to car-bohydrates. This was only because I experienced it firsthand.

One morning several years ago, after having enjoyed a few months of feeling wonderful, I woke up feeling lethargic with a headache and was extremely dazed and confused. Needless to say I was concerned, afraid that the wonderful new way I had been feeling was only temporary. I thought it had begun to wear off. For a few days after, I walked around quite perplexed, but feeling healthier each day.

Then, several days later while preparing dinner, I realized that I had inadvertently eaten canned peas that contained sugar! Following that, all of my previous doubts were permanently erased from my mind. Even after this experience, however, I still wanted to see the medical research concerning carbohydrates and addiction to further convince myself.

Sweetness Preference

First, we will review some of the earliest studies involving sweet-tasting foods. Next, we will look at those that included carbohydrate addiction. Studies throughout history have proved that overweight humans and animals eat more sweet-tasting food than those of normal weight.[16] The recorded enjoyment of sweet-tasting foods has also been linked to obesity.[17] These early studies laid the foundation for modern medical investigations into the reasons for sweetness preference, which has continued to be studied throughout the years.

For example, a 1989 study by Peter J. Rogers and John E. Blundell, published in *Physiology and Behavior*, involved two different tests on forty-four undergraduate volunteers of normal weight. Its purpose was to determine the effects of sweetness on food intake. Subjects were fed low-fat plain yogurt with four different sweeteners added. These included maltodextrin, glucose, and saccharin, which are all forms of sugar.

Participants were not told the purpose of the study. They were given a complimentary lunch, then unbeknownst to them were monitored. Those who were given the sweeter yogurt mixture ate more. The study concluded that "sweeteners stimulate appetite," promoting an increase in hunger and food intake.[18]

Erin I. Kleifield and Michael R. Lowe conducted a similar study in 1991. It showed that people who had recently lost weight preferred sweet tastes more than those who had kept their weight off for an extended period of time. The researchers concluded that "recent or ongoing weight loss enhances sweetness preferences and increases intake of sweet foods."[19] Taking it a step farther, Kleifield and Lowe also determined that long-term maintenance of weight loss may diminish one's preferences for sweets.

These studies and others involving sweetness preference have consistently found that even so-called normal people prefer sweet-tasting foods. One of the most startling notions researchers recently learned is that animals also prefer sweet foods. A 1993 study demonstrated that untrained rats strongly prefer carbohydrates, including sugars, starches, and maltodextrin, a type of sugar.[20] If an animal is able to make this distinction, imagine how intensely a food addict's body can crave carbohydrates.

Physiological Addiction

To explain the physiological reasons for these preferences, researchers have time and time again turned to animals. Most notably, a study involving rats proved that "enhancement of insulin secretion [takes place] in the early phase after a glucose load with food intake." This means that after eating a form of carbohydrate, more insulin was produced in the rats' bodies. As we have already discussed, this results in an increased production of serotonin.[21] Since our physiological makeup is similar to that of rats, it is safe to say that we experience the same process.

The physical cravings a food addict experiences were studied by medical researchers in an experiment conducted at the Massachusetts Institute of Technology.[22] Twenty-four obese people who claimed to crave carbohydrates were monitored during a four-week period.

Regular meals, designed to meet daily nutritional needs, were provided with no choice of food. A computerized vending machine monitored individual eating patterns between meals. Participants could choose between five high-protein and five high-carbohydrate snacks, each containing 165 to 179 calories.

The high-protein snacks were rarely chosen, while the foods high in carbohydrates were consumed at a significantly greater rate. Two individuals ate only carbohydrate-filled snacks. Most participants consumed approximately three to five carbohydrate snacks per day; however, one person ate ten and one-half carbohydrate snacks in one day.

When subjects were unknowingly given the amino acid tryptophan, several significantly decreased their carbohydrate snack intake. Researchers concluded that "some overweight people who claim to crave carbohydrate-rich foods actually do manifest cravings when given a choice between readily available, highly palatable carbohydrate and protein-rich snacks."[23] It was further concluded that obesity in some individuals may be related to disturbances in brain serotonin levels.[24]

This, along with the previously mentioned studies, proves that even the traditionally conservative medical profession has begun to recognize food addiction as a valid biological condition.

Drs. Kenneth G. Goodrick and John P. Foreyt, both with the Nutrition Research Clinic of the Department of Medicine at Baylor College of Medicine, discuss the addictive nature of food in their *Journal of the American Dietetic Association* article.[25] The doctors point out that behavioral treatments for obesity do not last "because they fail to address the addictive nature of eating" in a population they have labeled "nonpurging bulimics."[26] These people are defined as those suffering from uncontrollable binge eating.

Additional Research

In addition to these studies, doctors have consistently published books and articles that mention the addictive nature of carbohydrates. A few examples follow. It is important to note that the majority of the books including this information are not designed specifically for weight loss, but for healthy eating. Recognition of carbohydrate addiction has been slow in coming in the general public. How many food addicts do you know who read healthy-eating books? Most never do. They always go for the traditional diet books instead.

Dr. Samuel Homola, a natural medicine expert, points out that "just about everyone who is overweight eats too much carbohydrate, especially the refined variety."[27] He notes that one chocolate bar "contains as much sugar as a dozen apples. Yet, one apple will satisfy the appetite more readily than a dozen chocolate bars. This is one reason why very few people build up excessive fat stores by eating natural foods."[28]

Nutritional researcher Dr. Lendon Smith also recognizes sugar and other foods as being addictive, resulting in a "craving for the substance which becomes the daily reason for existing."[29] He further points out that "sudden withdrawal [from these substances] produces uncomfortable symptoms."[30]

The withdrawal from carbohydrates is also discussed in an article by Dr. Robert Lefever and Marie Shafe in *Employee Assistance.* They identify sugar and white flour as products that decrease the natural supply of neurotransmitters, including serotonin.

According to the article, "One actually becomes intoxicated by the sugar, white flour and other refined carbohydrates as they act like alcohol in the blood system and hypothalamus."[31] The authors also reinforce the notion that when insufficient amounts of neurotransmitters are produced, cravings and depression occur.[32]

Similarly, Dr. Larry B. Christensen says that eating carbohydrates increases the amount of brain serotonin in the bloodstream. This results in cravings for sweets when there is a serotonin deficiency.[33]

Fat Consumption

Still convinced that carbohydrates are not a problem for you? Then think about the amount of fat you eat. Some medical researchers believe that fat can be more addicting than carbohydrates. A consensus has yet to be reached, however. Adam Drewnoski, a nutritional researcher at the University of Michigan, points out that his research has shown most cravings to be fat-driven.[34]

Since fat contains more than twice as many calories as carbohydrates ounce per ounce, it saturates the body with an abundance of calories very quickly. According to Sarah Leibowitz, a Rockefeller University neuroscientist, a brain chemical called galanin may cause cravings for fat. In a test using rats, Dr. Leibowitz found that rats who craved fat had higher levels of galanin.[35]

Additionally, it was found that higher levels of galanin and neuropeptide Y, which controls carbohydrate intake, were present in genetically obese rats.[36] "They [the rats] may get a kind of double whammy when it comes to cravings," Dr. Leibowitz noted.[37]

What does all of this mean for you? It means that food addiction, though well hidden and slow in being recognized, is only just beginning to be seen as a medical affliction with physiological implications. For the first time ever, competent professionals are realizing that there are biological reasons for obesity and that willpower is not a factor in the struggle with weight loss. This means that without this knowledge you could not have stopped yourself from eating the things you did.

Those Who Disagree

Now, to be fair, we will point out a few of the opposing or misleading theories regarding the physical addiction to food. Some of these have received widespread media attention.

In *The Wellness Encyclopedia,* by the editors of the University of California, Berkeley, *Wellness Letter,* the craving of pleasurable foods is recognized. The effects of eating a meal high in carbohydrates are also described. The authors note that "some experiments during the last decade have found that a meal high in carbohydrates (whether sugars or starches) and low in protein may lead to a relaxed feeling, sleepiness, and decreased alertness by boosting the level of a brain neurotransmitter called serotonin."[38] Despite this, the authors are also quick to say that these symptoms do not qualify as an addiction.

Another theory, involving deprivation, has gained attention throughout the past decade. Psychological experts have studied for years why some people cannot seem to keep off or lose weight. Several have suggested that when individuals give themselves permission to eat anything and everything they want, they will eventually feel satisfied and begin to eat normally. This method may be effective for someone who is only psychologically addicted to food. For food addicts with the biological abnormalities we have described, however, this is a recipe for true physiological devastation. Their bodies would physically crave carbohydrates to a greater degree. Additionally, they would be forced to eat larger amounts of food to maintain the "status quo" their bodies have developed in order to produce a sufficient amount of serotonin. These addicts' bodies would constantly experience intense cravings for carbohydrates .

Similarly, a few years ago, the *Carbohydrate Addicts Diet* received national recognition. While the authors, Rachel and Richard F. Heller, recognized the addictive nature of carbohydrates, their solution was to eat them for only one hour a day. This was combined with two other meals low in carbohydrates. "The Reward Meal," as it was called, could consist of any food dieters wanted. The authors, however, did recommend that the meal be nutritionally balanced.

Limiting the number of times a day that individuals consumed carbohydrates, the authors believed, would decrease the intensity and recurrence of hunger and cravings. The key word here is "decrease." Why would anyone choose to live their lives with only half as much pain when none at all is necessary?

Another drawback to this diet is shown in one of the authors' own case studies. A woman in the book said she grocery shops specifically for her "Reward Meal." Isn't the point to stop obsessing about food completely? And for a true food addict, how long before sixty minutes turns into a full day? A week? A month? A year? A lifetime? For those truly addicted to food, this plan is similar to Russian roulette—you never know when the bullet will strike.

We wonder if these experts would tell an alcoholic to drink everything in sight, but only for an hour each day. It sounds ridiculous, doesn't it? Would you offer an alcoholic an unlimited supply of liquor, even if it were only for an hour a day? Of course not, and neither should a food addict be told to eat anything and everything desired. Theories such as these only help to strengthen the already powerful denial mechanism present in so many food addicts. You will read more about this later.

In line with this, a best-selling diet, *Sugar Busters!,* has recently acknowledged the existence of physical sugar addiction but advocates using wine, chocolate, nuts, pancakes, and even beer glaze in their meal plans. While this may work for those seeking gastronomical relief, for a food addict eating these substances will trigger overwhelming physical cravings, thus making it impossible to follow the diet plan.

With information like this provided to the general public, it is easy to see how the facts about food addiction are buried under a mound of misinformation. Who, after all, wants to admit that something as comforting as a chocolate chip cookie is as addictive for some people as alcohol is to alcoholics?

The Good News

How are you holding up after reading all of this information? Don't worry, it gets easier from here on. We know that it can be scary and overwhelming to discover these facts. We are sure your first thoughts are about all of the foods you think you will have to give up now that you know. But, did you think of all you will GAIN?

Imagine getting through a whole day without thinking about food, except at proper mealtimes. Think about eating a healthy, satisfying meal without feeling one ounce of guilt or shame. And how about never having to eat powdered, packaged diet food again to lose weight? Imagine being at a comfortable, healthy weight for your height, without starving yourself.

Think about the self-respect you will gain from knowing that you are not to blame for failed weight-loss attempts. And what about the immense feelings of relief that come from believing that, before now, you could not have stopped yourself from eating all that you have eaten?

Even greater than this, realize how much more energy and time you will have now that your life no longer revolves around food. You will have the time, stamina, and desire to do all of the things overeating took away. Isn't there a hobby, activity, or even a career that you used to do or have always wanted to try? Well, without food monopolizing your life, you will be able to do this. It will not happen overnight, but it will happen.

> Ten years ago, I wouldn't have been able to write a book, especially about something I did not even know existed. It was all I could do then to get out of bed each day. Though I've always wanted to write, my writing career got buried beneath my obsession with food. About twelve years ago, I made an attempt at a writing career, even getting an editorial published in a national magazine. The time and energy I spent eating, however, robbed me of my ability to pursue my career any further in the writing field.
>
> Nothing was as important to me as eating, and given the choice between eating or writing, *I always chose eating.* Gratefully, my life today is a lot different, and yours can be too.

What is it that you have neglected while eating? The logic about this goes something as follows: I do not have time for _____ anymore. (Fill in the blank.) Maybe you have even convinced yourself that _____ does not matter or that it is not important now that you are older.

> I told myself that writing was too hard for me to do on a daily basis and that I didn't like it enough. What I really meant was that I would rather have done something that was safer and easier so I would have more time to eat, though I didn't know it at the time.

How much time does eating and thinking about food take up in your life? Remember to include time spent watching television cooking shows, reading cookbooks, food shopping, figuring out how to hide snacks, planning meals, and preparing food. While some amount of time for several of these activities is necessary for survival, constant preoccupation with food is not.

No matter how you answered any of the questions asked in

this chapter, or how you feel right now, congratulate yourself for having read this far. Whether or not you believe it, you have shown a lot of courage for even buying this book, never mind reading through the second chapter.

Again, the only thing you need to do right now is to be willing to keep on reading. You do not have to worry about all of the food you think you cannot eat anymore. You do not need to concern yourself with what you can eat. For now, just keep reading and learning about food addiction. Read one chapter at a time and get from it the information that will help you. It is not possible to absorb the contents of this book immediately, nor should you try. Only concern yourself with reading this book in its entirety.

Chapters 3 and 4 are devoted to the new diet pills. You will learn how they work and the medical evidence surrounding them. Then, the dangers involved with these pills will be discussed.

Again, it is important for you to continue reading to have all of the information you need to make a clear, informed choice. You are worthy of that!

3

What about the Pills?

Take a pill, lose weight. Sounds great doesn't it? While the media has been focused on the fact that some diet drugs may help people lose weight, they have often neglected to point out that taking pills of any kind is replacing one addiction for another. The most common among these diet drugs, sibutramine (Meridia), dexfenfluramine (Redux), and fenfluramine and phentermine (Fen/Phen), have repeatedly gained widespread attention. But, as we now know, some of these drugs aren't as wonderful as we were first led to believe and others have their problems too.

In this chapter, we'll discuss the craze that surrounded the recalled diet pills (dexfenfluramine and fenfluramine) and examine the newer drug that was recently approved by the Food and Drug Administration (FDA)—Meridia. The historical discussion about the recalled diet pills reveals just how desperate food addicts needing relief can be. Keep in mind that there are people who, even today, would still take these diet pills despite the deadly risks. What does that say about the desperation food addicts experience?

Diet Pill Basics

Fen/Phen first gained widespread attention after the publication of several articles in the May 1992 issue of *Clinical Pharmacology and Therapeutics* by Dr. Michael Weintraub, an associate professor of community and preventative medicine of pharmacology and medicine at the University of Rochester School of Medicine and Dentistry. During his four-year study, Dr. Weintraub tested 121 people, ages eighteen to sixty years old, who were from 30 to 80 percent over their ideal body weights. Study participants were divided into two groups— those who took a Fen/Phen combination and those who were given a placebo with no medication. After about eight months, the group taking the medication lost an average of 15.9 percent of their initial weight while those taking the placebo lost 4.6 percent. While this may sound impressive, it is important to note that there were many additional findings that have not been as widely reported.

After stopping the medication, almost all of the study participants regained the weight they had lost during the experiment. Additionally, when dosage levels were doubled, twenty-five individuals either gained weight or stayed the same, while only eleven lost weight. These findings prove that without the pills, individuals experienced the same results dieters normally have—a 95 percent failure rate.

Let's look at these drugs. What could have been so bad about something that helped people lose weight? Before we answer that, it's important to understand exactly how these pills work.

Remember our discussion in chapter 2 about the brain chemical serotonin? Food addicts have low levels of this chemical, which predisposes them to overeat. Thus, raising one's serotonin level would promote weight loss. The best—yes, we said best—way to boost serotonin levels is through a healthy eating plan. There is no serotonin pill you can take to get that calm, happy feeling most food addicts crave.

The diet drugs fenfluramine (Pondimin) and dexfenfluramine (Redux)—which contain essentially the same active ingredient—enhance or stimulate serotonin activity in the brain. Although fenfluramine was FDA approved and was used before the 1992 publication of Dr. Weintraub's study, it was used rarely. Its use was mainly restricted to cases of life-threatening obesity, as the drug caused extreme drowsiness. Fenfluramine forces nerve cells to release serotonin, which triggers a feeling of satisfaction. Therefore, people feel full, but because serotonin also controls the body's mood and sleep feelings, taking fenfluramine also results in sleepiness.

To counteract fenfluramine's drowsy effects, phentermine, a mild amphetamine-like drug, also approved by the FDA, was introduced. And as shown in Dr. Weintraub's study, the combination—Fen/Phen—didn't put most people to sleep. In most cases, it perked them up.

"Fenfluramine takes the nerve cells and sort of beats them to make more serotonin," according to Dr. Michael Myers, medical director of Cerritos Weight Control and Medical Clinic. "It's like beating a horse. It speeds up for awhile, but it gets tired eventually. Later on, you start to get a depletion of serotonin. It could damage nerve cells."[1]

Dexfenfluramine (Redux) was approved by the FDA in 1996. Redux was on the market for only fifteen months when both it and fenfluramine (the Fen of Fen/Phen) were recalled.

Phentermine (the Phen in Fen/Phen) was not recalled. It has since then often been combined with the antidepressant Prozac, another drug that affects serotonin levels in the brain.

If you're like most food addicts, you may still be intrigued by the notion of a pill to help you lose weight. It seems so much simpler and, of course, easier, doesn't it?

Diet Pill Research

In a 1994 study documented in *The Journal of Pharmacology and Experimental Therapeutics*, monkeys given only four days of dexfenfluramine (Redux) showed major reductions of serotonin when their brains were examined seventeen months later.[2] Although it is true that these animals were given doses threefold higher than those recommended, they were exposed only to four days' worth of the drug. Would you be willing to risk permanent brain damage to lose weight?

Sadly, we know from experience that some people would consider taking the risk. Food addicts who are desperate and in pain are, most times, willing to do anything to ease their suffering and that includes risking physical harm to themselves. This was quite evident in a 1991 report on formerly obese people who had lost at least one hundred pounds. When questioned, 90 percent of these people said they would rather have a leg amputated or go blind than return to their former weight![3] Can you relate?

Maybe so, but weight loss does not require drastic measures. For 90 percent of food addicts who do not suffer from additional psychiatric or psychological afflictions, all that's needed is a healthy, balanced eating plan. While it may seem impossible now, the fact is a balanced food plan will control your physical cravings for food.

As Dr. Arthur Frank, medical director of the George Washington University Obesity Management Program, points out, all drugs did was tilt the odds toward success. He says they offered a "10 to 20 percent boost."[4] As he and others in the medical profession stress, what's needed most is a sensible diet and exercise program. Those who did choose to take diet pills still needed to follow a healthy eating plan and to be under the care of a doctor. In fact, many were probably given an eating plan similar to that outlined in this book. The important exception is that they weren't told to avoid carbohydrates. Information about this would have made a great difference in their success.

It's also important to remember that simply taking diet pills doesn't guarantee that you will remain thin. Remember the people in Dr. Weintraub's study? Even with double the dosage of Fen/Phen, the majority of them gained weight. As Dr. Kenneth G. Goodrick of Baylor College of Medicine pointed out in late 1996, "We had some patients gain weight while taking the medication, because it is possible to eat three cheesecakes on the medication."[5] Taking the pill didn't guarantee weight loss. They still had to do the work! At the same time, people who chose to take the diet pills were putting their lives in danger.

The only difference the pills made was in the rate at which individuals lost weight initially. The pills increased your metabolism so calories burned faster. But at what price? How many sleepless nights did these people have? The pills did not magically make them thin while they continued to eat whatever they wanted. Read that sentence again: the pills did not magically make them lose weight while they continued to eat whatever they wanted. Somewhere in the back of every food addict's mind is the hope that someday he or she will be able to eat everything and yet lose weight.

It is vital to remember that there is no magic wand. No supernatural force is going to come down from the sky and instantly remove all of your excess weight or take away your physical cravings. While a power greater than yourself may aid you on your path to recovery, you must be the one to take action. No one and nothing can magically take away your problems. There must be some work on your part. Unless you suffer from additional psychiatric problems that require medication, you can eliminate your physical cravings by avoiding your addictive substances. It really is that simple. While diet pills may increase your odds of weight loss by a small percentage, they also increase your chances of physical ailments and put your life at risk. After everything you've been through, do you really want to get involved in something else that may harm you? You deserve better.

Emotional Risks

While the physical risks of turning to pills of any kind are serious, the emotional risks are equally important. Compare it to alcoholism. If an alcoholic were given a pill to replace liquor, how long would it be before he or she took an extra pill when things got difficult? And, convinced that the pill helped him or her get through, how long before this person switches addictions?

What's different with a food addict? In our culture of bigger, better, and faster, it's only a matter of time before people wanting to lose weight take it upon themselves to increase their prescribed dosage. And when we're talking about messing with brain chemicals or using stimulants, there is great potential for deadly results.

The reality is that any drug designed to make people feel better has the potential to be addictive, if not physically, then emotionally. For long-suffering Americans, taking a pill is often much easier than actually working through problems. We have been conditioned to believe that little pills will help whatever ails us. But is that what's really in our best interest?

Don't think it could happen to you? Well, consider the words of James R. Winn, executive vice president of the Federation of State Medical Boards: "The long-term use of diet drugs is extremely controversial. There's a strong likelihood weight clinics will abuse these drugs." Winn warns that although the effects are milder than amphetamines, "the feeling of higher energy that Fen/Phen stirs can be habit-forming."[6] As an official of Ohio's medical board, William Schmidt knows firsthand just how addictive these diet drugs can be: "I have to tell you flat out that phentermine is abused. We've had a doctor lose his license because he became addicted to phentermine [the Phen in Fen/Phen], and others have been disciplined for overprescribing it."[7]

A New Pill

The FDA approved the use of sibutramine, commonly known as Meridia, in late 1997. Though it works differently from Fen/Phen and Redux, the drug also affects brain chemistry. Similar to the fenfluramine in Fen/Phen, Meridia boosts brain levels of serotonin, although in a different way. The former diet pills stimulated the production of brain chemicals, while Meridia slows the breakdown of neurotransmitters. Theoretically, the slightly elevated brain chemical levels appear to be less dangerous than the high ones caused by Fen/Phen and Redux, although the drug's effects have only been studied for one year.

As with any drug, Meridia is not without side effects. Some of the more serious ones include an increase in blood pressure and heart rate, both of which are already commonly high in obese people who don't take diet pills. Dry mouth, headaches, and constipation are also listed among the "lesser" side effects.

Initially, the FDA's advisory committee recommended against the approval of Meridia due to the risk of high blood pressure, potentially increasing this risk for those who consider using it. As with any drug, a possible side effect of Meridia is physical dependency, as stated in the manufacturer's own advertising. Choosing to take this, or any other drug, to lose weight, may be a way of simply replacing one addiction for another. Even worse, you may end up having two addictions to deal with rather than the one you originally had. Does that seem worth the risk to you? Before answering this question, remember that you still must eat a well-balanced diet while taking the diet pills.

You don't have to put your life at risk or become dependent on yet another substance. Simply follow what is outlined in this book and your life will change. While it is important to be medically evaluated by a licensed professional to determine whether you have further emotional problems, get all of the facts before making any major decisions.

A substantial amount of medical evidence supports the food addiction theory. Now you've seen how the diet drugs work to alter the very brain chemical that you can manipulate with a healthy eating plan. So, how do you feel? Think about your life right now. Are you happy? How's your health? Do you feel completely overwhelmed by life? Is your eating out of control? Is it hard for you to move around? Do you always seem to be tired? If you answered yes to even just one question, it's vital that you continue reading and learning. For now, we'd like to remind you what you are actually moving away from. A discussion of the medical consequences of obesity follows.

The Consequences of Obesity

Known as "Simple Obesity" in the International Classification of Diseases, obesity is classified as a general medical condition. It does not, however, appear in the *Diagnostic and Statistical Manual of Mental Disorders,* fourth edition (DSM-IV) because obesity has not been clearly linked with a psychological or behavioral syndrome. In the *Johns Hopkins Family Health Book,* men are defined as obese "when fat accounts for 25 percent of total body weight," and women are defined as obese "when fat accounts for 30 percent of body weight."[8] There is still great confusion and little agreement about obesity in the world. What's clear are the medical consequences of obesity.

Obesity plays a significant role in the formation of a disease called atherosclerosis, commonly known as hardening of the arteries. This disease predisposes people to coronary heart disease, abnormalities of the electrical functioning of the heart, and the formation of clots. Additionally, diabetes and hypertension are two other major diseases in which atherosclerosis plays an important role.

Obese people face more serious complications from hypertension. Strokes occur more frequently among the obese, which usually results in paralysis, or even death. With obesity, the death rate from heart disease, primarily caused by blood vessel disease, is approximately 50 percent higher in men and 75 percent higher in women than in the normal-weight population. Likelihood of cerebral hemorrhage or stroke is about 60 percent higher than normal, and the presence of kidney disease appears to be approximately 100 percent higher.

Recent studies also indicate that there is an increased risk of breast and endometrial cancer (cancer of the inner lining of the uterus) in obese individuals. Cancer of the liver and gallbladder is 70 percent more frequent in obese men and 110 percent more frequent in obese women than it is among their normal-weighted counterparts. Incidence of cancer of the intestines and rectum is 15 percent higher, and cancer of the female organs is 20 percent higher. Additionally, when compared with the normal-weight population, incidence of diabetes is 300 percent higher in people who are obese. Cirrhosis of the liver is 150 percent higher; appendicitis, 120 percent; hernia and intestinal obstruction, 50 percent higher; gallstones, 100 percent; complications during pregnancy, 60 percent; and cancer of the pancreas, 50 percent higher in obese women.

Obviously, obesity needs to be taken more seriously. In the back of your mind, are you thinking of looking into what kind of diet drugs are available? Are you actually excited by the prospect of taking a pill to lose weight? If so, you are like most food addicts. In chapter 7, you will learn about the various ways your mind plays tricks on you. But, for now, simply realize that whether or not you decide to look into taking diet pills, you now know another way. There is a completely natural solution to your overwhelming physical cravings for food. You no longer have to continue harming yourself. You do have a choice.

For most long-suffering food addicts, the side effects of diet drugs may seem a small price to pay for thin bodies. Maybe, but what's the difference between being addicted to food or to drugs? Is that what you really want? To trade one addiction for another? The emotional and physical ramifications of drug dependence and food addiction are nearly identical, so what are you really changing?

The choice is completely yours—a natural, lifetime cure or a two-dollar-a-day drug habit. Which do you think drug manufacturers want you to pick? If you're still unsure, continue reading. Your life may depend on it!

4

Just How Dangerous Are Diet Pills?

Imagine having a device attached to your waist that is connected to a catheter in your chest which constantly pumps medicine into your lungs. The pump electronically regulates the medicine and must be packed in ice every four to six hours. The medicine must be mixed each day, and the dressing on your chest catheter must be changed every three days. All this for the low price of $3,800 per month.

Sounds horrible, doesn't it? Well, those who took the Fen/Phen and Redux diet pills increased their chances of developing primary pulmonary hypertension by as much as 30 percent. This is a sometimes fatal disease that damages the heart when not enough oxygen is pumped to it. If you were lucky enough to survive, you would have a choice: the pump or a dangerous lung transplant. An August 28, 1997 article in *The New England Journal of Medicine* reported that a twenty-nine-year-old woman who took Fen/Phen for twenty-three days died of pulmonary hypertension. How much weight do you think she had time to lose before she died?

While primary pulmonary hypertension was perhaps the most serious side effect of these diet pills, there were others that are just as disturbing. But before we discuss them, we would like to present an overview of the FDA's approval process as related to the diet drugs.

FDA Approval

Shouldn't drugs approved by the FDA be safe? Although both fenfluramine and phentermine were each approved, the combination of the two was never reviewed for approval by the FDA. Therefore, Fen/Phen, as it was prescribed across the country, was not technically approved by the FDA.

While Redux, which has the chemical properties of fenfluramine with the same active ingredient, was approved by the FDA on April 29, 1996, it was not the first time drug manufacturers sought approval. A year earlier when Redux was up for approval, the FDA advisory committee rejected the drug by a five-to-three vote due to questions of safety. Following that meeting, an FDA official reopened the discussion after some committee members had left. Since there was no longer a quorum, a new meeting was called for two months later in November. By that time, the members opposed to the drug were absent, as the FDA's meeting just happened to coincide with an international neuroscience conference in San Diego.

If that's not enough, a high-profile board member of the drug's manufacturer, Interneuron, was sent to the FDA's meeting, leading to charges that Redux was moved through improperly in a high-pressure lobbying effort. While the drug won approval at the FDA's second meeting in November, it was by a one-vote margin. "We weighed the idea of putting off the decision for several months until those experts could be there," said FDA official Dr. James Bilstad. "Since the committee had heard their presentations before and were given transcripts, we decided that we had the benefit of their comments on the issues. It was a judgment call." Though the committee's decision wasn't legally binding to him, after several months, FDA Commissioner David Kessler gave his approval, but with conditions. The drug manufacturers were required to do follow-up testing in the form of clinical studies, to monitor the drug's side effects.[1]

Additionally, the FDA imposed a very tight restriction on the drug. Redux had to be marketed and prescribed for use only by patients who were life-threateningly obese. That means only people who were at least 20 percent to 30 percent over-weight should have been using the drug, for a limited time, in conjunction with a diet and exercise program. After evaluating the results of nearly three hundred patients' heart tests, the FDA issued a statement on September 15, 1997, urging individuals to stop taking Fen/Phen and Redux. The test results showed that 92 of the 291 people studied had damaged heart valves even though they had no symptoms. Following that, the FDA requested that drug manufacturers voluntarily recall their products. Both companies agreed.

The Payoff

With more than half of America's adult population being overweight—that's upwards of fifty-eight million people—any drug promising to ease the burden of this many people can cause quite a stir. Both Fen/Phen and Redux certainly did that. Not only did they hold their own in the pharmaceutical market, after only a short time, they nearly dominated it. In 1996, Fen/Phen was the second fastest growing drug, making $191 million that year for its manufacturer. Over the three-year period since the Fen/Phen study was reported in *Chemical Pharmacology and Therapeutics,* prescriptions for the drugs rose from 60,000 to about 1.1 million. In the first five months after its introduction, doctors wrote 1.2 million prescriptions for Redux, with sales totaling more than $20 million a month. Wyeth-Ayerst, the makers of Redux, estimated that more than two million people took the drug during its fifteen months of existence. Couple that with the four million who have used fenfluramine (Pondimin)—since 1973, with most being in recent years. There seemed to be no stopping the diet-pill revolution. As David Crossen, of Montgomery Securities in San Francisco, said of Redux in early 1997, "What we have here is probably the fastest launch of any drug in the history of the pharmaceutical industry. Our projection is that this product will hit $1 billion in sales in five years."[2]

Luckily for everyone, Crossen's projections proved untrue.

Yet, with profits like these, there was certainly ample incentive for manufacturers to push their products. While Redux was approved on the condition that it only be used in cases of "morbid obesity," American Home Products, the drug's marketer, launched an aggressive campaign aimed not only at obesity specialists, but to general practitioners, psychiatrists, internists, cardiologists, and gynecologists, all of whom may not have been as knowledgeable about the drug's side effects or treatment plans.

While American Home spokespeople said the drug was used by only 250 doctors "sparingly" and that more than 90 percent of those patients were morbidly obese, the numbers didn't quite add up. With sales totaling more than $20 million a month, there was certainly room for debate. In the first three months alone, Redux salespeople visited 140,000 doctors to "educate" them about the new drug. Who's kidding whom?[3]

As weight-loss expert Dr. Michael Myers pointed out in late 1996, "They hand it [Fen/Phen] out like cheap Halloween candy. It goes down real easily that evening, but the next morning you get the bellyache. We haven't even begun to experience the bellyache.

"The perception in the lay community, and unfortunately for the most part in the physician community, is that these drugs are a miracle answer," Dr. Myers says. "They don't understand that Fen/Phen is really only an adjunct to diet modification, behavior modification and exercise." Morton Maxwell, head of the obesity clinic at the University of California Los Angeles agreed: "A very large proportion of people are using [Redux and similar drugs] for cosmetic weight loss. It's really scary."[4]

The Scams

Just how scary was it? Take into consideration Dr. Peitr Hitzig. With a flashy Internet Web site, Dr. Hitzig promised patients hope with Fen/Phen. "Uncontrollable urges to eat disappear. Cravings for junk food vanish. The tendency to overeat ceases," are the promises advertised, complete with flashy graphics and a philosophical comparison to Hippocrates. Touting Fen/Phen as the answer to everything from Gulf War Syndrome to chemical hypersensitivity, Dr. Hitzig urged his Web site's visitors to contact him for the drugs. And, if you couldn't make it to his Timonium, Maryland office? No need to worry. He was prepared to work around that. "Although we greatly prefer to see everybody in the office when the program is started, we can make exceptions if there are strong reasons that you can't make it to the office," his material proclaimed.

Strong reasons? Here's a man, a Harvard-educated physician, who was offering to prescribe Fen/Phen without ever even seeing his patient! How much did Dr. Hitzig charge? According to his own literature, "The charge for the first six months of treatments is only $1,154. During these six months we will teach you the basic fundamentals of the Fen/Phen program. You will learn how to regulate your own dose. No matter how many times you have to call, there will be no further charges. We expect a down payment before the first visit of $350. We can make arrangements if there is financial necessity. After the first six months, the charge will be only $327 every six months to continue the treatment."

Consider two very important facts when reading the doctor's message. First, the medication itself sold for about $60 to $70 a month. What was the additional $125 per month for? Second, what Dr. Hitzig conveniently "forgot" to mention was that initial medical studies proved that the risk of lung disease rose if patients used the drugs beyond three months. And here was Dr. Hitzig promising to give patients a year's supply. Ask yourself, who's getting rich here?

Dr. Hitzig's literature boasted "treating patients in 33 states on five continents, within five provinces of Canada and in eight European countries." You do the math! Sadly, Dr. Hitzig was not alone. Several other doctors also promoted the weight-loss drugs via the Internet, with one California doctor promising increased metabolism, reduced hunger, and safe weight loss at $65 for the first visit with a $20 charge for the medication. Charges for additional visits were $35.

If you were looking for a bargain, one physician on the Internet, Dr. Ben Krentzman, a Culver City, California, general practitioner who came out of retirement in 1993 to promote Fen/Phen, promised to provide you with Fen/Phen rather than Redux. "Redux wholesales for three times the cost of Pondimin (fenfluramine). So, if you insist on Redux, I will get it for you, and charge you three times what I would for people using Pondimin. Since the medicines are identical I will bow to the wishes of my patients," his material stated. Proclaiming Fen/Phen safer than aspirin or driving a car, the doctor pointed out that he would prescribe the drugs for you even if you were thin. "I see many people who are in extreme discomfort after years of fighting to lose 15 to 20 pounds. I have given up judging people's emotions about their weight," his material stated. "I have seen people 120 pounds overweight who were only slightly upset by their weight. And I have seen people who were 15 pounds overweight having anxiety attacks about their inability to get rid of their excess weight. So I don't judge people, any longer, on how upset they are about their weight."

If a medical doctor wasn't comfortable making judgment calls, would you want this person to be your physician? Keep in mind that if you had decided to take Fen/Phen from Dr. Krentzman, you would have been required to sign a release stating that the dangers of the drugs had been explained to you, "both verbally and in writing. Then I treat them like any other overweight person starting with me," he says.

Chances are that with more than three hundred patients and nearly one hundred thousand visitors to his Science of Obesity and Weight Control Web site, Dr. Krentzman isn't worried about what the FDA thinks. His advice to people wanting to lose weight remains the same: take the pills instead of worrying about diet and exercise. He says, "Dieting and exercise without Fen/Phen doesn't keep people slender, so why should they work with Fen/Phen?"

What about these doctors and their flashy Web sites after the drug recall? Unbelievably, as of late 1997, neither had addressed the voluntary recall. Dr. Krentzman's Web site remained outdated while Dr. Hitzig changed the name of his. Now known as the Fen/Phen Crisis Center, the Web site tells patients not to worry about the risks of the pills. Proclaiming himself the "primary practitioner and father of the Fen/Phen protocol," Dr. Hitzig tells his patients that they "typically receive half of the Fen/Phen dosage . . . therefore, the risks of Fen/Phen are not typically caused by the protocol itself, but by lack of education on the part of doctors who prescribe a single, fixed dosage for all patients." Once again, there is, however, no direct mention of the recall in his Web site.

The Popularity

Thankfully, these two doctors hold a minority view, but the Internet wasn't the only place where you could have gotten these pills. Most national diet centers like Jenny Craig and Nutri/System incorporated the drugs into their programs. A half-page advertisement in early 1997 for Nutri/System's new RX Program advertised, "We have Fen/Phen. No food purchase necessary."

And there was no stopping the pills' attractiveness. One weight-loss clinic in Independence, Missouri, had about four thousand clients on the drugs, while nearly 70 percent of the one thousand members of the American Society of Bariatric Physicians, doctors who are interested in obesity treatment, at one time or another had prescribed the drugs.[5] Compare that figure with the 30 percent who prescribed it before 1992.

Even more disturbing was the growth of unscrupulous weight-loss centers, know as pill mills. "I'm seeing a trend toward less-than-ethical treatment in storefront weight-loss programs and a flurry of misleading advertising designed to lure overweight people," said Dr. Richard Joseph, chairman of the ethics committee of the American Society of Bariatric Physicians.[6]

At one DuPage County clinic in Illinois, for example, a forty-six-year-old woman, Kathy, from Naperville was shocked by her experience. At a walk-in clinic, patients were seen on a first-come-first-serve basis. The forty dollar cost, which included a month's supply of Fen/Phen, was payable only in cash. Checks, credit cards, or health insurance claims were not accepted. "I filled out a standard health questionnaire and waited two hours before a technician called my name," she said. "He took my blood pressure and pulse and gave me a vitamin B-12 shot. He said I had to go back to the waiting room and wait for somebody else to call me and I would be given a month's supply of pills. I thought, 'This is weird; he's not a doctor.' A half-hour later a woman called my name. She wasn't a doctor either. She said I had to drink lots of water with the pills, which she said were appetite suppressants. She said if I felt funny after taking them to call. I asked her what she meant by funny. She said to call if I got light-headed or if I felt my heart beating faster."[7]

Thankfully, Kathy refused the pills and quickly left the clinic, but she may have been in the minority. How many other people do you think accepted the pills? Take David, forty-two, of Naperville, Illinois. He visited the same clinic as Kathy. His blood pressure registered a few points too high to qualify him for the pills. But he didn't have to worry. A woman who identified herself as a nutritionist had the answer. "She said to go to a doc-in-the-box type office and get a diuretic prescription [a water pill to eliminate excess fluid in the body] so my blood pressure would drop enough for me to come back and get the Fen/Phen. I expected to be seen by a physician. I wasn't. I just didn't trust that place."[8]

What about people who saw their family physicians and asked for the drug. If your doctor didn't believe in the diet pills, you couldn't have gotten them, right? Maybe. Maybe not. The demand for the drugs was so powerful that even physicians had lost control over them. Take Dr. Susan Wickes, a family physician with the Mayo Clinic in Scottsdale, Arizona. "Some of the patients are saying, 'If you don't give it to me, I'll go down the street and get it at another clinic,'" she said. "So sometimes I cautiously prescribe it, because I would prefer to continue working with my patients."[9] Sounds like blackmail to us.

The Side Effects

If all of this doesn't scare you, let's talk about the side effects of these diet pills. Primary pulmonary hypertension is perhaps the most dangerous side effect of both Fen/Phen and Redux. When the FDA approved Redux, research showed that the risk of developing primary pulmonary hypertension was nine times higher on the drug.

Medical studies later proved otherwise. The risk of developing the disorder was actually thirty times higher in people who used the pills for longer than three months. Recent studies suggest that the number may even be greater. That's quite a difference from the initial reports.

And, as Joanne P. Ikeda, cooperative extension nutritional education specialist with the University of California, points out, "This statistic assumes that every single patient with primary pulmonary hypertension is diagnosed, and that every single case diagnosed is reported by the doctor to the European Drug Agency, correctly connected to the use of the diet pill, and entered into a government file.

"There is very good reason to believe that fewer than 10 percent of cases are successfully counted through this whole process. The diagnosis of primary pulmonary hypertension is very difficult—a heart catherization must be done. The only symptom may be shortness of breath—very common in fat people. Death could be the next symptom," she said.[10]

No one really knows yet how high the risk of getting primary pulmonary hypertension is. The drug manufacturers' own news release about the increased danger of developing the disease says, "Primary pulmonary hypertension is a serious disorder with a four-year mortality rate of 45 percent."

The news release also points out yet another serious possible side effect of the diet pills—brain damage. Buried in the second to last paragraph, it says, "FDA is emphasizing that all appetite-suppressing drugs should be taken only under careful medical supervision. In addition to concerns about pulmonary hypertension, questions also have been raised about studies showing long-term changes in the brains of animals. The relevance of these animal findings to humans is not known."[11]

In a study conducted by Dr. George Ricaurte of Johns Hopkins Medical Institute, it was proved that fenfluramine significantly and perhaps permanently damaged brain cells in baboons. And, though he's unsure about similar effects in humans, he is worried. "There is every reason to be concerned that it may [damage human brain cells]," he said. "Once you destroy them, [they] don't have the potential to recover or regenerate. So these are not short-term effects that we're noticing one or two days after the drug treatment; these are long-lasting effects."[12]

While even today, drug manufacturers are quick to point out that there is no medical evidence to support the theory that Fen/Phen and Redux create long-term brain damage, there are documented cases of short-term difficulties. According to nutritionist Joanne P. Ikeda, "In several cases people have suffered from a complete loss of short-term memory. This does tend to go away for the most part after stopping the drugs. However, the question of permanent impairment is not answered—there are no long-term studies of memory function."[13]

Those Affected

Still not convinced? Read on. One woman, Phyllis Ojeda, became depressed and forgetful after taking Fen/Phen for the first time. "I was saying the alphabet to my grandson, and I couldn't remember what 'd' was. That scared me to death," she said. According to California nurse Lynne Nieto, Phyllis's experience is not unique. "One patient in Huntington Beach stated she suffered from insomnia, she felt she was jumping out of her skin, irritability," she said. "She went to the emergency room and was referred to a psychiatrist."[14]

Then there's Betty Moore of Long Beach, California, a sixty-four-year-old nurse. "In the beginning, it was like a little miniature amphetamine," she says of Fen/Phen. "I definitely got a lift." But it didn't stop there for her: "I was irritable and quick to anger. I was very emotional. Everything seemed more important than it was. A couple of times I went off it, and I really didn't want to move."[15] And when she stopped using the drug, her depression remained. Though Margaret Herman of Long Beach, California, is satisfied with the results of Fen/Phen, even she was quick to admit suffering side effects. "It does affect your head," she said. "I was forgetful. Your thoughts are kind of scattered. You're peppy, but you can't direct it."[16]

Yet another serious side effect of the drugs was the risk of "serotonin syndrome," a chemical overdose that can cause tremors, seizures, and even organ failure. This could have occurred when the pills were taken with Prozac or other antidepressants. As Kirk Mills, an expert on drug interactions at the Detroit Poison Control Center says, "I don't know if we're going to come across another drug with as much potential to cause serotonin syndrome as this one [Redux]." New evidence has shown that as many as 30 percent of diet-pill users could develop abnormalities in their heart valves. Changes in the shape of the valves could eventually lead to death.[17]

Other possible side effects from Fen/Phen and Redux included severe diarrhea, extreme mood swings, shortness of breath, racing heart, irritability, depression, impotence, loss of sexual appetite, headaches, dry mouth, drowsiness, insomnia, fatigue, vivid dreams, hallucinations, anxiety, and manic-depressive reactions.

The Alternatives

Now that you've read about the dangers of these pills, are you considering the now-popular herbal Fen/Phen or perhaps the new Phen/Pro combination or another "miracle" drug? If so, think about all that you have just read. Then, consider that herbal Fen/Phen bears little resemblance to its chemical counterpart. The pills are simply a mixture of herbs known to be stimulants. To date, thirty-eight deaths have been associated with ephedra, the herbal stimulant in herbal Fen/Phen.[18]

Some experts consider herbal Fen/Phen to be more dangerous than Redux. Dr. Arthur Frank, medical director of the

George Washington University Obesity Management Program points out, "These herbal preparations are very impure. You could have some guy grinding up cigar butts in his garage and packaging them as supplements and you'd never know it."[19] Is that what you want for yourself?

As for the Phen/Pro combination, Prozac operates in the same manner as the now-recalled fenfluramine. While some "experts" will tell you that there are less side effects with Prozac, remember that, as with the now-recalled Fen/Phen, no one really knows what happens when two drugs are combined together and taken over a long period of time.

As Dr. Frank notes, no controlled studies demonstrating the effectiveness of this drug combination have been done. "It's an outrage, the kind of irresponsible thing that should not be done," he said. Dr. Frank also notes that Prozac has not been approved by the FDA as an obesity drug.[20]

As Dr. Lewis J. Rubin, chief of pulmonary and critical-care medicine at the University of Maryland and an expert on the effects of the diet pills, points out, "There's no data on any of this stuff."[21] Do you want to be the drug manufacturer's next test case? This question is worth asking about the newer diet drug, Meridia. Though there have yet to be documented cases, those taking this drug run the risk of experiencing serious side effects which include high blood pressure and increased heart rate. For overweight people who already experience these health problems, these pills may result in deadly consequences. Keep in mind that this drug, like those before it, was initially denied FDA approval only to gain it after a year's worth of testing. Would you bet your life on this amount of research? That's what you may be doing if you choose this or any other diet drug.

As we have told you, there is a completely natural alternative to these diet pills that will take away your physical cravings for food without *any* of the dangerous side effects. So, what do you have to lose? Some weight?

Why not read on and discover this natural alternative before you rush out to get any type of pill. It may not be as difficult as you think, and it may save your life. Do you really want to risk permanently injuring yourself? If not, turn the page.

5

Are YOU a Food Addict?

Unsure about whether or not you are addicted to food? If you are like most food addicts, at this point you are trying to convince yourself that carbohydrates are not a problem for you. You want to believe that you are not one of those people we are talking about in this book. Do not make a final decision until you take the quiz in this chapter.

Before you begin, though, there are a few things you should keep in mind while taking the quiz. First, and most important, be rigorously honest. If you answer maybe to any question, it counts as a yes. Unless you are absolutely certain that you have never done or felt like what is asked of you, answer yes. And do not worry about what other people will think; you are the only one whose opinion matters. Remember, your answers are your own business. If you decide to share them with someone, that is your choice, but if you prefer to keep them personal, that is your right.

The Quiz

Now it is time to find out if you really are a food addict. Just check yes or no after the following questions. Go with your first instinct. Good luck!

1. Do you think about food a good majority of the time?
   _____ yes _____ no

2. Are you ever afraid there will not be enough food?
   ____ yes ____ no

3. Sometimes do you feel driven to eat? ____ yes ____ no

4. Do you physically crave certain foods? ____ yes ____ no

5. Have you ever lied about how much you have eaten?
   ____ yes ____ no

6. As time goes by, does your eating get worse?
   ____ yes ____ no

7. Do you hide or sneak food from others? ____ yes ____ no

8. Is it sometimes hard for you to concentrate because you
   are thinking about food? ____ yes ____ no

9. Have you ever used food to change your mood? That is,
   to make you happy or because you are bored.
   ____ yes ____ no

10. Do you start a diet only to find yourself pigging out a
    short time later? ____ yes ____ no

11. Do you either frequently weigh yourself or completely
    avoid stepping on the scale? ____ yes ____ no

12. When in public, do you either consciously avoid food
    areas or spend all of your time there? ____ yes ____ no

13. Is it hard for you to understand how someone can
    throw away food? ____ yes ____ no

14. When you have dieted in the past, have you ever
    experienced headaches, depression, or weakness?
    ____ yes ____ no

15. Do you ever feel out of control when eating?
    ____ yes ____ no

16. Has your body size ever affected your ability to partici-
    pate in certain activities? ____ yes ____ no

17. Have you ever fantasized about or looked forward to
    eating? ____ yes ____ no

18. Do you sometimes eat a lot more than you planned?
    ____ yes ____ no

19. When you have not eaten your favorite foods in a while,
    do you feel angry or depressed? ____ yes ____ no

20. Have you ever abused anyone—physically or emotionally—because of your eating behavior? ____ yes ____ no

21. Are there times when you cannot remember what you have eaten, or that you have blacked out? ____ yes ____ no

22. Do you have unique eating habits or rituals? (e.g., only eating three kernels of popcorn at a time)? ____ yes ____ no

23. Have you ever eaten before you went out for a meal so you would not eat a lot in front of others? ____ yes ____ no

24. At any given time, can you name most, if not all, of the food in your house? ____ yes ____ no

25. Does it seem as if food is the only thing in your life that never lets you down? ____ yes ____ no

The Results

If you answered yes to at least ten quiz questions, you may be a food addict. To learn more about your addiction, ask yourself these questions: How bad are your cravings? How often do you have them? Is food ruling your life? For how long have you been bingeing? Just how distracted by food are you? How much do you eat before going out for a meal? How often do you use food to change your mood?

These types of questions will help you determine just how serious your problem is. If you are like most food addicts, your life is totally unmanageable and revolves around food. It is not necessary, however, for your symptoms to be that pronounced. You may be one of the lucky ones who is able to recover without ever hitting bottom. In other words, you may not have to suffer as much as many do if you are able to recognize your symptoms early enough.

Another factor in evaluating your answers lies within the questions themselves. Answering yes to questions about cravings, blackouts, or mood changes, for example, is more characteristic of a true food addict than lying about food. Both are done by those who are addicted. Some food addicts, especially those living alone, may not have any reason to lie about what they have eaten. They do, however, experience cravings or mood changes.

It is important to remember that not all food addicts do everything mentioned. Some may sneak food while others would not dream of doing so. One food addict may step on the scale religiously each day, while another will avoid it at all costs. Some may spend hours fantasizing about food, while others might be too busy eating to daydream about food. Consequently, there is no one foolproof quiz for determining food addiction. This quiz is an attempt to make you aware of the characteristics of food addiction so that you can decide for yourself.

The Realization

One of the most helpful things I did was to write out a history of my eating life. I started with my earliest memories of food, including ones my parents had told me about, and worked my way through to the present.

With each incident I remembered, I wrote exactly what I ate, how I felt before, during, and after eating, and the way I acted throughout the entire experience. For example, I discovered that before eating I was usually excited, anxious, and happy. Though I didn't realize it at the time, I learned that I fantasized endlessly before eating, creating a dreamlike state. The most exciting part for me was the first few minutes of eating. I felt euphoric as I looked at the food laid out in front of me.

As I continued eating, however, I began to worry that there wouldn't be enough food to fill me. I started planning what I would make next, though, most times, I had enough for twenty people; then, I began to eat as fast as I could. I wanted to make sure I had enough time to make something else to eat. I felt nervous, worried, and anxious.

About halfway through, the guilt and shame would begin to wash over me. Deep inside, I didn't want to hurt myself, yet I couldn't stop. When I finally finished, I felt powerless, humiliated, sad, angry, and depressed. The "hangover" was always so much more painful than the good taste of the food, yet I couldn't stop myself from eating it.

After reading several of these incidents I had written about, it struck me quite hard. If I could have changed my behavior at that time, I would have. But, because I didn't know about my addiction or how to help myself, I was powerless to change. Thankfully, my life changed dramatically the minute I discovered this concept.

Now, think about yourself. After eating a lot of sugary foods, do you fall asleep almost immediately or do you yell at a family member or friend? What usually happens immediately before you start eating? Do you plan exactly what you will eat, or is it a spontaneous decision? Compare the amount you planned to eat with what you actually ate. How do you feel while you are eating? Are you excited? happy? upset? depressed? Whatever you feel, write it down. When doing this, remember that it is possible, even common, to feel conflicting feelings—such as happiness and anger—at the same time. (Do not "edit" your feelings; simply write them down.) What about when you finish eating? Do you eat more? How do you feel? Think about your physical symptoms. Do you have an especially difficult time getting up the morning after a late-night binge? Are you in more physical pain—backache, sore feet, upset stomach—than usual? And what about your mood? Do you wake up depressed or angry, scared, guilty, or ashamed?

No matter how awful you think it is, just write. By letting the memories flow freely, you are allowing yourself a chance to be completely honest. This will help you determine the extent of your addiction. When you are finally finished, put your writing away for at least a few hours, if not a full day, before reviewing it. If you are able, the most effective way of reading it is in one sitting, completely undisturbed. This will give you a chance to view your eating history as a whole, instead of in bits and pieces.

Feelings

Most food addicts, due to years of escape with food, have lost touch with their emotions. Some are so far gone that they are unable to even put a name to what they are feeling. Feelings are different from judgments. A judgment is always made in your mind. "I'm fine," for example, is a statement about yourself, not about what you are feeling. Other judgments include good, bad, dishonest, upset, disrespected, misunderstood, put upon, and judged.

The key difference between feelings and judgments is that feelings take place inside your gut, while judgments come from your mind. Most feelings are extensions of the "basic four"—sad, mad, glad, or scared—often used by counselors to help children describe what they are feeling.

Saying you feel "misunderstood," for example, might really mean that you feel frustrated, angry, or sad. When you say misunderstood, you are making a judgment about what the other person is thinking, not about what you are feeling. Feelings mention only what YOU are experiencing, not what you believe another person is THINKING.

When you have finished reading your eating history, take some time to think about it. Are there similarities in the types of food you eat regularly? What about the times of day or events leading up to your binges? Noticing these patterns is invaluable to understanding your addiction. They will be especially helpful when you begin to develop a personalized food plan in chapter 11.

Right now, just begin to notice your patterns, most important, your food choices. Being a food addict is no reason to be ashamed. In the same way that people with cancer are not blamed for their illness, food addicts should not be blamed for theirs. Both are based on biological malfunctions, not personal choices.

Keep reminding yourself that *you did not choose to be a food addict.* It is a disease that you cannot control, but you can learn to live a happy, sane life despite your affliction.

Before making a final decision about whether or not you are a food addict, read the next chapter. This will give you a fair shot at reaching an educated conclusion about your condition. You deserve that much. You are worthy of a life free from obsessing about food. Even more than that, by following these suggestions, it is possible to stop craving food. So, read on and find out how!

6

Who's Addicted to Food?

How did I get this disease? What caused it? When will it go away? These are probably a few of the many questions running through your mind at this point. Let's start with how you got this disease. As with any relatively new discovery, there are many questions and few concrete answers about food addiction. Several theories, however, have been developed over the past decade or so.

One of the more recent conclusions about the cause of food addiction involves the amount of yeast in our bodies. While everyone's body contains a certain amount of yeast, known as "*Candida albicans*," an overgrowth of it can stimulate sugar cravings.[1] Since yeast feeds on sugar, an overgrowth of it is believed to cause cravings for the substance.

What would cause an overgrowth of yeast in your body? The answers might surprise you. Stress, hormonal changes, lowered immunity, sugar, and long-term antibiotic use are all believed to contribute to yeast overgrowth.[2] Therefore, the more sugar you eat, the more yeast you produce, the more sugar you crave. Think about your own life for a second. Does this seem to make sense, judging from your experiences?

I know that when I first heard about this theory, I was shocked. As a child, I suffered from chronic bronchitis, which resulted in the use of antibiotics at least twice a year, usually much more. Though I sometimes wonder about the association of yeast with sugar cravings, I cannot deny that it seems to add up in my case.

Dysfunctional Society

A less physiological theory states that all addictions—food, sex, money, alcohol, drug, and so on—are adaptations to a dysfunctional society.[3] Addictions are viewed as "mood changers" sought to meet individuals' needs that are not being adequately met in the "social, economic, and spiritual fabric of our culture."[4] Some of those needs include belonging and intimacy, meaning, purpose, fun, creative play, consistency, and self-acceptance.[5]

The authors of this theory point out that "addictive ways of thinking and behaving are actually reinforced by many aspects of our culture."[6] When we take this assumption into consideration, using food as an example, it seems highly plausible. Consider the introduction of the "drive-through window" at fast-food restaurants a few decades ago. With this innovation, food addicts can quickly and effortlessly get their binge foods without the embarrassment of leaving the car.

Or, what about all of the ready-to-eat food available today? Can this be considered yet another way that society is feeding the food addicts' addiction? Even those not addicted to food are freed from the time it takes to prepare a meal, allowing them more energy to pursue their own addictions.

If we enlarge this idea to include other addictions, namely money, work, and power, an even stronger argument can be made supporting this theory. Who are the heroes we look up to? Celebrities, financial moguls, and industry leaders, all of whom must work excessively to achieve their success. Ten- and twelve-hour workdays are lauded as sure roads to success, failing to take into account other aspects of people's lives.

Hypoglycemia

Still another theory on the origins of food addiction is that hypoglycemia causes sugar cravings. Hypoglycemia is a state in which your body cells are consistently low in fuel due to abnormal glucose metabolism. It is concluded to be a factor in causing your blood sugar level to drop well below normal.[7] Eating a great deal of refined carbohydrates may cause an excessive amount of insulin to be released into your system, causing the pancreas to malfunction.[8]

According to this theory, some foods are quickly digested, such as those containing refined carbohydrates and alcohol. They are released into the bloodstream immediately, causing your body to be excessively efficient in removing sugar from your bloodstream. This would, in turn, cause a craving for more carbohydrates.[9]

A reasonable amount of medical evidence supports this notion. And we are convinced that hypoglycemia contributes to food addiction in some people. But the devastating physical deterioration of true food addiction cannot be explained solely on the basis of insulin release. If this were the sole reason food addicts craved food, what would account for the extraordinary amount of pleasure a food addict gets from eating? That can only be explained by including the neurological aspects of a person's physiology.

Dieting

Continuous dieting has also been linked to the development of a food addiction. As we mentioned earlier, several medical studies have proved that dieting causes your body to prefer sweet tastes and results in a cycle of deprivation.[10] However, advocates of this theory fail to fully address the neurological aspects of food addiction.

Again, we are confident that these theories play a role in food addiction, but are not solely responsible for its origination.

Predisposition

Finally, two other theories attribute a predisposition to addictive disease as the reason for food addiction. One mentions scientific evidence that our bodies are programmed to respond to sweets from birth. It points out that "hard-wired circuitry from the tongue directly to the brain makes us enjoy sweet things."[11] The other theory says that food addicts experience a significant mood-alteration through carbohydrate use, similar to the "high" an alcoholic gets from the first drink.[12] Both theories involve a predisposition in some humans as the reason for food addiction.

Again, some scientific as well as personal data we have collected supports the conclusions made in both theories. This alone, however, cannot explain the origins of food addiction. What can then?

Our Theory

When taken as a whole, several of these theories combined accurately explain the origin of the disease of food addiction. We agree that nearly all food addicts are predisposed to their disease. We are also confident that it is both a physiological and psychological predisposition.

In the same way that some family members pass down their sicknesses, such as diabetes or heart malfunctions, food addiction is inherited. This is not to say that family members are to blame. They were simply innocent carriers of the disease and not the cause of it.

> In my family and in that of other food addicts, some of whom you will hear about in this book, addictive disease was present in different forms. Both of my grandfathers were alcoholics, as well as several other family members. Additionally, food was always used as a reward or comfort during my growing years. Thus I was predisposed to seek food as a psychological comfort at an early age.
>
> Physiologically, due to the strong presence of addictive disease in my family, my biological makeup predisposed me for a physical addiction. This was triggered early by my food use, resulting in both a physiological and psychological addiction.

Think about your own family. Is anyone an alcoholic? Include those already deceased who you may not have known, as the physiological tendencies could have been passed down. Is anyone in your family a drug addict? This includes relatives who use prescription or nonprescription drugs, especially diet pills. How about food addiction? This includes family members with anorexic or bulimic tendencies, as well. Does anyone in your family smoke? Some believe nicotine to be the most addictive drug available. Other addictions include gambling, shopping, television, sex, or codependency—addiction to other people. Is there someone in your family who suffers from any of these? While these may seem "less physical" than an addiction to drugs, alcohol, food, or nicotine, they are just as serious, merely in different ways.

"Who really cares if my grandmother was a compulsive shopper?" you may ask. You should care! Chances are that it is affecting you today, whether or not you realize it. How? There are certain attitudes that go along with any type of addiction. These are usually passed down unknowingly from generation to generation. Your grandmother, then, most likely passed addictive behaviors down to your father who, in turn, gave them to you.

Remarkably, all of this is done unconsciously without, in most cases, any intent of harm. For example, let us just say that your grandmother was a compulsive shopper. It may be true that your father did not use shopping in the same way she did—as an escape or a way to deal with his feelings. It is very possible, even likely, that he found another substance to use in the same way your grandmother used shopping. He was taught, by example, to handle his problems this way.

We have seen and heard of many food addicts who are, at first, puzzled about the presence of any addictions in their families. After giving it careful consideration, however, they become enlightened to the possibilities. Maybe his father was considered a "big eater" but in reality was a food addict. Perhaps her mother had "a condition" for which she needed to take pills constantly. Grandfather only went to the racetrack a couple of times a week, and Aunt Jennie surely could not help it that she simply liked shoes so much her closet was overflowing with more than fifty pair.

And what about little Suzie? Surely she would gain weight soon, after all, eighty-five pounds is not that unhealthy. Then, there is big brother Bob who just cannot seem to stay away from women. He sometimes had as many as five sexual partners at once. What about the cousins who cannot seem to stop watching television? And their parents—Mother who schedules her life around soap operas and Father who would rather die than miss a hockey game?

And the Jones sisters? One sister continues to stay with her physically and mentally abusive husband even though he nearly killed her two weeks ago, and the other smokes like a chimney. They couldn't have an addiction, or could they?

These are only a few examples of the many addictions present in society. Did you recognize any from your own family? Considering that denial is ingrained in families after years of living with an addiction, this is no small task.

In the next chapter, we will explain how difficult it is to recognize denial. When reading that, consider how hard it would be to break through generations of denial. That is what you are trying to do—take everything that you grew up believing was "normal" and rethink it.

It was not normal for your father to come home so drunk that you had to help him to bed. It was not normal for your mother to need six diet pills a day to maintain her trim figure. Twelve hours of television viewing is not a normal daily occurrence. Betting twice as much money as they have or shopping until every single credit card is over the limit is not normal either.

These are not "normal" experiences, even though you may have come to believe that they were during your childhood. The addicts in the family had to convince you that their activities were acceptable in order to continue using their substances. Just as denial is present in your disease and it took hard work for you to admit your addiction, your family members also struggle with denial.

Addictive Patterns

The point here is to recognize the addictive patterns in your family. This will help you answer questions about where your addiction came from. And you will be able to see how powerless you were over developing your addiction.

Well-known medical authority Dr. Bernie S. Siegel says in his healing lectures that parents are not to blame for dysfunction or addiction because they had parents. These parents had the same afflictions, and so did their parents, and so on. Siegel's problem is with "Adam" and "Eve" because they started it all!

While at first this may seem silly, it is worth discussing. When you first discover addictive patterns in your family, it may be tempting to admonish or at least point out the problem to those involved. This is not necessarily the most effective means of dealing with the situation. Remember, these people most likely suffer from addictions in the same way that you do.

How did it feel when someone pointed out how much weight you had gained or how tight your clothes were? What about when well-meaning friends would mention the newest miracle diet on the market? Or when your spouse lovingly "pinched an inch" on your stomach? Think about the shame you felt when diet foods or exercise equipment was brought into the house as a motivational ploy to get you to lose weight. It hurt, didn't it?

It was very painful whenever my family members or friends tried to coax me into losing weight. Even though all of these gestures were done completely with love, I still felt embarrassed, ashamed, humiliated, and desperate. I wanted to lose weight so badly, yet nothing seemed to work. I blamed myself, with each failure believing myself to be more hopeless than the last.

The point is, I knew I had a problem; I just did not know how to solve it. For a long time, quite frankly, I was not willing to work at making myself well. Food was so important in my life that I did not even want to consider giving it up, until it got too painful to keep on eating.

By confronting the addicts in your life at this time, you risk making a bad situation even worse. The addicts may not be ready to deal with their problem. By trying to force them to recognize their affliction, you may alienate them, thus closing the door on any productive help you may be able to provide in the future.

Other People

Other people's addictions are none of your business. You have enough dealing with yourself. You do not need to be worrying about anyone else's problems, no matter how serious you believe them to be. You are responsible for yourself in the same way that other addicts are responsible for themselves.

Effective ways to deal with such situations will be discussed in a later chapter, which will include healthy ways to state your feelings and needs. Until then, just concern yourself with your own addiction. You have enough to handle.

It is also worth mentioning that by concerning yourself with other people's problems, you are taking the focus off your own. This gives you the perfect excuse not to deal with your food addiction. If your spouse has a drinking problem, how can you be expected to deal with your food addiction? That problem has to be taken care of first, right?

Wrong! Spouses, older children, parents, siblings, friends, co-workers, and grandparents, to name a few, are all capable of living their own lives without interference from you. Contrary to what you may believe, they do not need your constant input in order to survive. It is time to stop concerning yourself with other people and take care of yourself. Use that energy to accomplish amazing things in your own life.

While parents with small children may be considering themselves exempt from the above information, they are not. Recovering from an addiction benefits everyone around you, especially those closest to you. It may be more challenging for those with small children to make time for themselves to recover from their addictions. It is, however, by no means an excuse for inaction.

Use your imagination to find the time you need. Find a baby-sitter for a few hours a week if you cannot do what needs to be done when the children are around. If you cannot afford a baby-sitter, try to arrange a barter system with other parents in your area and take turns caring for each other's children.

Still not convinced that you can squeeze any extra time into your schedule? Look harder! What about the time you spend at night watching television or talking on the phone? How about getting up ten minutes earlier each morning or going to bed a little later? If possible, hire someone to do a chore that will provide you with extra time to devote to yourself. As financial guru Tony Robbins says in his self-help tapes, "There's always a way if you are committed." Are you committed to recovering, or is this just a little something you thought you would try?

It does take some time to recover from food addiction. There is no magic cure. As much as you do not want to believe it, there is no pill or drink that will instantly make you thin. It takes a concerted effort on your part to recover from your addiction, but it is by no means impossible. You are capable of doing it, but the question is, are you willing to make the effort? Before answering that question, think about the reasons you picked up this book initially.

> I know from personal experience how painful the disease of food addiction is. I especially remember the self-hatred I felt when I had eaten more than I ever thought one human being could in one sitting. Or the humiliation I suffered when still another pair of pants wouldn't fit anymore no matter how much I tugged at them while lying on the bed. And the desperate loneliness I felt from being locked in a world without any hope of ever leaving.
>
> Taken by themselves, these memories are enough to make me want to follow my program. When put together, however, the pain of these experiences still affects me today. I never want to feel anything like that again, and thankfully, since I began this program, I haven't.

Remember the last diet you tried? What happened? How successful were you? And your last binge? How did it end? Were you crying? Or maybe the pain was so great that you were not even able to shed any tears. Think about all of the times you wished you had gone to the beach or out dancing but were too ashamed of your body. And the cravings you experience on a daily basis. Do you want to continue to live like this? The choice is yours. If you want things to change, you have to make time to change them. It is that simple. It is important to begin thinking of where you will get the time to work your recovery program. It is not, however, vital that you map out your entire schedule for the next three years.

Think only about today. Tomorrow will take care of itself. We know you have heard that before, but have you ever really thought about it? If you are like most food addicts, you never honestly thought about a lot of things, except food and eating. What this means is that if you live your life in a healthy, productive way today, then tomorrow will be the same. You have set up a pattern or habit for constructive living.

Healthy Habits

Contrary to what you may believe, all habits are not bad or negative. There are many healthy, constructive habits that you can develop to help you recover from your food addiction. One, which we discussed earlier, is the habit of weighing and measuring your food. There is nothing harmful about that. Weighing and measuring may save your life by helping you to heal from your food addiction.

Some other productive habits include exercising, eating properly, writing about your feelings in a journal, and telling your spouse you love him or her. You already have many healthy habits that you probably do not consider to be habits. These include showering or bathing regularly, brushing your teeth, washing your clothes, and cleaning your house. Even going to work is a constructive habit. With all of these habits you already have, getting into the routine of being in recovery should be easy, right?

Let's look at some of your more destructive habits. Do you always eat while you are watching television? Are there certain shows that you absolutely will not miss? Do you have favorite foods that go along with them?

For me it was afternoon soap operas and popcorn. Each weekday, I would rush home to watch my soap operas and eat my microwavable popcorn. I always made it a point to eat the popcorn during *As the World Turns,* my favorite of the four soap operas I watched. That was the highlight of my day—being with the two things I loved most in this world.

The thing I never even considered after getting into recovery was that I was still in the habit of wanting popcorn or another food whenever I watched television. The first time I sat down to watch a show, I remember feeling as if something was missing. I was not quite sure what. Since I had such a strong habit of eating while watching television, it was an entirely new experience to sit through a show without any food.

It was also one of the most rewarding feelings I ever experienced. I was not driven to get up every five minutes or during every commercial to run for the refrigerator. I was able to actually concentrate on and enjoy a television show instead of obsessing about food or worrying who might catch me eating. What a freedom not to worry about the crumbs or mess I was making. I did not have to try to eat as much as I could as fast as I could while still trying to concentrate on the television show!

Another similar habit I had was eating popcorn every single time I went to the movies. During each movie, I had at least a medium, if not a large, bucket of popcorn, smothered in butter and salt, and a medium diet soda. Just as important as the food was the timing. I liked to eat my popcorn in the dark where no one could see me. I usually tried to time it perfectly to have the food exactly when the movie started, most times sitting with it uneaten until the darkness came.

Many times I went to the movies solely for the popcorn, not caring what show was playing. I was only concerned with the popcorn I could eat in the safety of the darkness. Sometimes I did not even remember what the movie was about, but I was always able to recall the luscious taste of the popcorn.

Can you relate to any of these experiences? What habits have you developed concerning food? Is there a certain food you absolutely must have every day? Do you honestly believe you will not make it through the day without eating one particular food? And what about your activities? Are there some things you could not imagine doing if one kind of food was not involved?

Think hard about the habits you have developed over the years. This will help you recognize your "danger times" where food is concerned. Each one of us has certain times of the day, week, month, or year that are particularly difficult to deal with. These are the times when we are most likely to turn to food because that is how we have always dealt with these situations.

What about you? Maybe your danger times have nothing to do with television. Perhaps they involve special times during the night. I have heard many food addicts tell about night being their most dangerous time. Many admitted to waking up at 2:00 or 3:00 A.M. to eat when no one else was awake. Does this sound familiar?

> Another danger time for me involved work. Many years ago as an editorial assistant for a weekly newspaper, I was the only employee in the office on Saturdays due to my school schedule. During this time, all I could think about was eating as I was trying to work. I even went so far as to rummage through my co-workers' desks to find food. Being there alone gave me the freedom to eat whatever I wanted without anyone knowing.

Have you had similar experiences? We have heard of people bingeing only when they went out to dinner to "celebrate" not having to cook. These people were able, for the most part, to diet whenever they did not go out to eat. To them, dining at a restaurant was a license to binge. It is worth noting that many of these people, as their addiction grew more serious, drastically increased the number of times they went out to eat.

Whatever habits you have, it is important to notice them.

Write them down so you do not forget. If you are still convinced that you do not have any, write down your eating schedule for one week. Note the times you eat, what you eat, and what you are doing while you are eating. This will help you to see any eating patterns you may have developed.

When trying to break these habits, always be gentle with yourself. Consider that it takes at least twenty-one days to form new routines. Think about how long you have been doing these things. They are not just going to disappear overnight. So be kind to yourself.

Try not to overwhelm yourself with thoughts about the information in this chapter. Yes, it is helpful for you to be aware of the addictions present in your family. And of course you need to understand your eating behaviors, but be careful not to use this as an excuse. Too much analyzation can lead to paralyzation in working your program.

Try to be satisfied with the things you do remember instead of dwelling on those you have forgotten or cannot understand. As you will learn in the next chapter, an outstanding characteristic of any addict is intellectualization. If you continue to devote all of your energy to contemplating the origins of your addiction, you will have none left to devote to your recovery. And make no mistake, recovery from food addiction should be your main goal.

Distractions

While discussing ways in which food addicts sabotage themselves, it is worth mentioning that distraction is one of the major ways people use to subconsciously confuse themselves into inaction. A food addict's battle cry is, "I am confused." By resorting to a confused state of mind, a food addict can delay recovery indefinitely. It is much easier to remain bewildered than to actually take action to recover.

Symptoms of using distraction to avoid recovery include constant analysis of healing methods, criticism of recovery concepts, procrastination with other so-called more important issues, and avoidance of the topic entirely.

Analysis leaves no room for open-mindedness, which is an

essential ingredient to recovery. When food addicts constantly analyze their addiction, the problem is kept entirely in their minds, safely tucked far away in an unreachable corner of the brain. This is similar to continually putting something on your "to do" list but never quite doing it.

Likewise, constant criticism of recovery concepts will also prevent action. In the food addict's mind, finding the flaws in anything provides a ready-made excuse for lack of mobility.

Then, there is procrastination. Do the words "I will start my diet on Monday" sound familiar? What about waiting until "the first of the year" or "after the holidays"? By procrastinating, food addicts give themselves the perfect excuse to eat everything in sight today. Think about how many diets you said you were going to start. What was the first thing you did after you made the decision? Go out for pizza or ice cream? Or, even better, go shopping?

> I always made a habit of stopping at the grocery store to get my favorite foods the day before I planned to start a diet. By doing this, I accomplished two things. The first, and most obvious, thing I did was to give myself permission to eat anything and everything in sight. On days before I started diets, I could "legally" binge. I did not have to feel ashamed or guilty about anything I ate because I knew that I was going to do something about it tomorrow.
>
> The second thing I accomplished, though I was unaware of it at the time, was to sabotage my dieting efforts. I filled the house with enough junk food for an entire month. When the ill-fated day to begin dieting arrived, I told myself there was too much food in the house for me to even consider such a feat. How could I let all of this food go to waste when there were people starving in the world?
>
> My procrastination for that day turned into at least a week, if not a month, usually resulting in more weight gained. That is the funny thing about procrastination—it is progressive in the same way the disease of food addiction is. The more I avoided

doing something, the harder it was to actually accomplish it. It never, ever got easier, only more difficult.

Just as hidden and cunning for most food addicts is the idea of dealing with other more important issues before tackling their food problem. Many food addicts believe that their lives must be in perfect order for them to finally take action on their food issues. When is the last time your life was perfect? That is exactly the point: there will always be another crisis to deal with, so it will never be the right time to recover from food addiction.

It works something like this: having other problems to handle gives addicts an excuse to eat. They believe they don't have enough time to work a recovery program. They are, after all, too busy handling other problems in their lives. When food addicts deal with their addiction, the other problems in life seem to be more easily managed, not the reverse.

And then there are the addicts who refuse to even discuss the topic of food addiction. In the addict's mind, if the problem is not discussed, then it does not exist. This means that no action must be taken.

While this may seem to be the most obvious form of distraction, it is often hidden beneath a mound of denial. A person who denies having a food addiction will often appear to have his or her life together. The person looks perfect on the outside but is really desperately unhappy inside. The difficulty here lies in the addict's convincing portrayal of his or her so-called happiness. Most people will not even realize the person is in pain. He or she appears too happy to be worrying about such issues as food and weight. Friends and family members, therefore, avoid the subject. In this case, the addict has created the illusion of a perfect world. This ensures the complete avoidance of the topic of food addiction.

This brief overview of distraction methods is not a complete summary of every characteristic present in all food addicts. As you progress in your recovery, you may find others not mentioned here. Each person, being a product of individual life experiences, will have different food-addiction characteristics.

No two food addicts are exactly the same. This information is especially meaningful during the early phase of recovery. The temptation to compare progress is very strong. As we discussed earlier, "terminal uniqueness" can be a tempting excuse for an addict to avoid recovery.

Equally enticing can be the desire to conform to others in recovery. Keep in mind that your friend or co-worker who is following this plan with you will have different results and experiences than you. Some may be the same, but many will be quite distinctive. Neither is wrong.

Perfectionism

The reason we mention this is to put to rest the perfectionist nature found in most addicts. There is no perfect way to recover from food addiction. The concepts of right and wrong should not even be a consideration, though they may be for many.

> In the early days of my recovery, I constantly compared myself to other food addicts, wondering if I was doing things right. I lived in constant fear that one wrong move would destroy all of the progress I had made. I honestly believed that if I made even one small mistake, I would be right back to where I had been before.
>
> After a little while, I learned that making some mistakes was a healthy thing to do. Making mistakes meant that I was, at the very least, trying new things, which is a sure sign of growth. Since I was starting to like myself more than I had before, mistakes no longer caused deep humiliation. Before, when I had done something I thought was wrong, it meant that I was wrong. Now, I recognize that I can make many mistakes without them affecting my self-worth.

Have you ever thought about mistakes before? How do you think of them? Are they a reflection on your entire worth or simply wonderful learning experiences? For many food addicts, due to stubbornness, complete recovery requires their making mistakes in the program. We have heard countless stories of people who, after devastating relapses, have returned with a renewed commitment to abstinence. Making a mistake turned out to be a valuable learning experience.

What about you? Are there mistakes you've made that have helped you to grow? They do not necessarily have to involve food for you to understand how mistakes work in your life. Think about the times in your life when you have learned the most. Did they not, in one way or another, involve a mistake?

> A big learning experience for me, though it took a while to realize, was being stopped for speeding in Liberty, New York. The police officer had been following me on the highway for several miles. I had not noticed him because I was too busy trying to reach for my roast beef sandwich. He clocked my speed at well over seventy-five miles per hour. I didn't even know I was speeding. I was too concerned with getting my lunch!
>
> From this, I learned how distracted by food I could become. At the moment when I was looking for the sandwich in the cooler, nothing was more important, including watching the road. Had I been an alcoholic, I would have been arrested on the spot. Food addicts do not get arrested for driving under the influence of their drug. Their actions, however, may cause just as much harm as that of someone driving while intoxicated. Since sugar, flour, and caffeine affect my ability to function normally, my perception is altered in much the same way an alcoholic's is when drinking.
>
> Today, my recovery plan includes not eating while I am driving. Though the foods I eat are not as intoxicating as those I once did, my attention to them is still considerable enough to cause a significant distraction.

According to Dr. Robert Lefever and Marie Shafe, "One actually becomes intoxicated by the sugar, white flour and other refined carbohydrates as they act as alcohol in the blood system and hypothalamus."[13] We remind you of this simply to reinforce the notion that food addiction is as serious as alcoholism. Society still has a long way to go in acceptance of this.

We know some of the concepts introduced in this chapter may be difficult to accept, but at least be willing to give them a fair chance. Your life depends on that. Millions of people die each year from food addiction. Death certificates, however, neglect to mention the disease by its proper name.

Several years ago, we heard of a five-hundred-pound man who was planning to admit himself to a food-addiction treatment hospital. He died the night before he was scheduled to be admitted. We are certain that his death certificate did not list food addiction as the cause of death. We hope you will use this story in the way it is intended—to show you how serious the disease of food addiction really is. People actually die from this disease. Our hope is that you are open-minded enough to prevent yourself from being yet another victim of this insidious disease. While some people die from this disease, others are reborn into a life they never imagined possible.

7

I'm Not Like Those People

By now, if you truly are a food addict, you are trying to convince yourself that you are different, that your problem is not serious. You would like to believe that your life is just fine. And you are telling yourself that, even if you do decide to take diet pills, the things we've talked about won't happen to you.

For the first several months after I had heard about food addiction, I tried desperately to convince myself that I was different from the other people I had met. Yes, I weighed more than three hundred pounds and constantly thought about food. But the rest of my life appeared to be in good shape, didn't it?

The key word in that sentence is "appeared." On the outside, I looked happy and well-adjusted. In reality, I was secretly stuffing my pain down my throat, desperately trying to understand why I could not lose weight. I spent a good majority of my time and energy trying to convince everyone, myself most of all, that I did not have a problem. Yet, my life was falling apart.

Ten years ago, I would have told you that my life was as wonderful as I wanted others to believe . . . as long as I did not think about it too much. Most times, however, I was just pretending so they wouldn't discover my food problem. Yet, part of me honestly believed that I had a wonderful life and that nothing was wrong with me. Another part, however, knew how desperately unhappy I was.

What about you? Is your life as wonderful as you would like others to believe? Are you just pretending so they will not discover your food problem?

Many food addicts report hiding their true feelings from other people. This is due to one of the most prevalent symptoms of food addiction—denial. As with any other addiction, denial is a major obstacle most, if not all, food addicts face. Denial about food addiction occurs because addicts either don't understand or don't accept the true characteristics and nature of the disease.

Denial

This is not to say that food addicts are purposely dishonest or of weak moral character. Denial is the brain's mechanism for protecting a person from events or truths that are too painful to deal with at the present moment. In some cases, denial has served as a lifesaving device for people, especially when involving incest. For the most part, however, denial for those addicted can be deadly.

Denial explains how a New York man can end up weighing more than 1,000 pounds. Or how a 588-pound European model can proclaim that fatness is a family trait and "truly has nothing to do with what I eat."[1] While it is obvious to you that these people most likely have eating problems, it is not to them. That is the essence of denial—everyone but the person involved is aware of the problem.

After you finished writing your eating history, were you surprised at how much food you actually ate? Or by the number of dieting attempts you had made? Did you realize that you had hidden food that many times? How important had eating become to you?

All of these things illustrate how strong the denial mechanism is in humans. It impairs a food addict's judgment and results in self-delusion that perpetuates a self-destructive pattern. Denial is an addict's way of pretending the addiction doesn't exist. This brings the person even deeper into addiction.

At 328 pounds, I had convinced myself of several things. First, that eating candy or sweets did not really make me gain weight. I thought that I did not look that bad, and certainly not like I weighed more than 300 pounds. And I believed that I did not really eat a lot.

What I didn't realize then was that I had a habit of looking at myself in the mirror from only the neck up. Very rarely did I see a full-length reflection of myself. And, when I did, I usually looked away quickly, pretending I hadn't seen anything. Since I hardly ever let anyone take pictures of me, I really had no idea what I looked like.

Though I knew from the pain in my feet and the size-forty-eight jeans I wore that I was overweight, I had no idea what I looked like at 328 pounds. I simply thought of myself as "pleasantly plump," not grotesquely overweight as was the case. While my denial protected me from the painful reality, it also allowed me to continue overeating without taking responsibility for my actions.

In other words, if my food addiction didn't exist, if I wasn't that overweight, then I didn't have to do anything to help myself. In my denial, I could continue doing the one thing I most wanted to do—eat. If I admitted my actual size to myself, then I would have to change. My denial kept me sick and nearly killed me.

Does any of this sound familiar to you? Is it hard for you to continue reading? If so, your denial may be acting up, trying to get you to put this book down so that your life can remain just as it is. Is that what you really want?

Denial is a powerful psychological defense that food addicts unknowingly use to protect themselves. A description of the various types of denial present in addicts follows.

Types of Denial

One of the most basic forms of denial is known as "simple denial." This is the notion that something is not so when in reality it is. Believing that eating high-calorie foods will not make you gain weight, for example, is a form of simple denial. Some other examples include being certain that your size-eight clothes will still fit even though you weigh two hundred pounds; knowing that the dozen cookies you just ate will not affect your diet; and believing that taking diet pills doesn't present any health complications. The food addict is unaware of the dishonesty involved in this form of denial. These are things that, at the time, the person honestly believes to be true, making it even more hazardous.

The next type of denial is called "minimizing." This is when the food addict will admit there is a problem, but only to a small extent. A four-hundred-pound man, for example, may believe that he has a "small weight problem" instead of the serious one he does. Saying that you have not eaten much food when you have binged twice is another example of minimizing.

Do you believe that your eating is all your spouse's fault? Or maybe your mother's, father's, your best friend's, or children's fault? If so, you may be suffering from the third type of denial known as "blaming." With this form of denial, the addict acknowledges the problem but blames it on someone or something else. This puts the responsibility for the problem on someone else. How many times have you blamed Thanksgiving, Christmas, New Year's, or Easter for your eating? Maybe it's the malfunctioning car, or the disobedient dog, or your small house, or simply boredom. By blaming, it is impossible for addicts to deal with the problem, which allows them to keep right on eating. Understand now how the thinking goes?

Similarly, "rationalizing" is providing alibis, excuses, justifications, and explanations for the addict's behavior. As with blaming, the behavior itself is not denied. Instead, an inaccurate explanation of the reasons is offered. "I only eat because I am bored," is a common rationalization. Others include eating because you are nervous, tired, angry, or stressed, and one of the most common among pregnant women—"I am eating for two."

"Intellectualizing" is another type of denial that involves theorizing instead of dealing with the emotional elements of food addiction. People who intellectualize read everything there is to read about eating disorders and may "know" they have a problem, but they do not feel the pain involved. The know-it-all who will talk for hours about the theories of food addiction without a trace of emotion or feeling is an example of someone who is intellectualizing.

Two other forms of denial are "diversion" and "hostility." Both of these involve shifting the focus from food addiction to other areas. With diversion, the food addict avoids discussing any threatening topics by changing the subject. The hostility type, on the other hand, avoids the food-addiction issue with anger or irritability. Both are very effective ways of making other people back off from the subject.

Finally, the last type of denial is known as "defiance." This is when the food addict is able to manage the anxiety behavior and masquerade as self-confident and reliable. People experiencing this form of denial are thought to be pillars of society. They usually are highly successful in their careers or appear to have a wonderful family life. In reality, they are desperately unhappy about their food addiction.

Some of these people may even try to convince you that they accept themselves at their weight. They want you to believe they are happy with their lives, though they may be extremely overweight. People in the defiance form of denial, whether knowingly or not, appear on the surface to "defy" the usual characteristics of addiction. Instead, they suffer in private, behind closed doors.

Do any of these sound familiar to you? Because denial is such a powerful mechanism, you may not fully believe you fit into any of these categories. You may, however, experience a strong reaction to one or more of the descriptions. Did you feel uncomfortable when you read any of them? Usually when we have a strong reaction to something—negative or positive—it means that we are touched on some level of ourselves, consciously or subconsciously. If you felt an unusually strong reaction to any of this material, chances are you suffer from that particular denial mechanism.

Managing Denial

Dealing with denial can be very overwhelming, even frightening. It is a good idea not to try and tackle everything at once. For instance, if you honestly believe that you tend to rationalize, begin to notice the ways in which you do this. With any form of denial, the greatest weapon you have is awareness. By being aware, you are breaking through the mechanism that works to keep you in your addiction. That is why writing out an eating history is helpful. If you have been as accurate as possible with your eating history, you probably learned some new things. Maybe you did not know you ate so much or that you acted the way you did after eating. Whatever it was, it can help you break through any denial you may be in regarding your addiction.

Remember, denial is a symptom of your disease, not a moral deficiency. If you had cancer or multiple sclerosis, you would have headaches, dizziness, or lack of muscle control. Instead you have a biological disease with both physical and psychological symptoms. A December 1992 study reported in *The New England Journal of Medicine* showed that obese people failed to lose weight after eating a diet reported to be low in calories. This was due to discrepancies in their reported food intake and their amount of physical activity.[2] Researchers concluded that obese subjects who had a history of failed dieting attempts "misreported their actual food intake and physical activity."[3] Additionally, the people in the study who reported less hunger and more restraint showed a greater degree of misreporting.[4] This illustrates how powerful the denial mechanism can be. The people who thought they ate the least were actually misreporting their food the most!

Society and Food

Another important element contributing to food addicts' denial is the societal attitudes surrounding food. While it is easy for people to realize that heroin is dangerous, a cream puff is a different story. It seems so harmless, and oh, the taste! Food has been used throughout history as a way to comfort the sick "feed a cold," show love, and provide relief from stress. Think about the messages the media give us on a daily basis. How often do we see a mother baking cookies or brownies for her family to prove her love for them? Now advertisers also make showing love "quick and easy" with microwavable products that take only minutes. What about the soup commercials where food is presented as a "cure-all" for a child's cold or an adult's heartache?

This attitude is not confined solely to the media either. What is the first thing we send children away at college or family members in the service? When a child cries, what do we reach for first to provide comfort? What do we use to help celebrate birthdays, holidays, and other special occasions? The answer is, of course, food. In our society food is considered to be good, a sort of reward we deserve for living another year or celebrating the birth of Christ. Can you even imagine a holiday without cookies, cake, or some other sweet dessert? Most people cannot.

> I wish I had a dime for every time someone asked me how I am able to go without eating sugar or flour. When a person first hears about my addiction, they act as if I should be given a sympathy card. "You don't eat cookies? How do you do that?" are the shocked questions I am asked. Sometimes I am treated as if I come from another planet. Even people who eat healthy—so I have been told—are allowed to have "just one" cookie now and then, right?

Our society has created certain attitudes about food that are widespread and powerful, even spilling over into people's religious ceremonies and beliefs. When Christians take communion, what represents the body of Christ? At Passover, what do Jewish people use to represent their religious commitments? When two people are joined in marriage, what is used to symbolize their joining during the reception? Again, the answer is food. Even the biblical downfall of man was shown by using food. After all, what did Eve give Adam? Food! With attitudes as powerful as these, it is easy to see how psychological and physiological dependencies are perpetuated. Not even our magazine shelves are safe. A quick look at *Writer's Market 1996* shows that the total combined circulation of food and drink magazines, not including diet food publications, is more than 4.5 million!

These examples are not presented so you will blame society for your food addiction. *No one can force you to eat anything you do not want to,* and that includes society, religious organizations, advertisers, magazine publishers, and grandmothers.

With that said, we would like to point out one last example of how denial works. Many food addicts believe that they are different from others or unique with their disease. This concept, often called "terminal uniqueness," serves to separate the food addict from others and perpetuate denial. The thinking goes something like this: "If I am different from others, then I am too sick to be helped, so I can continue to eat whatever I want."

As with the other forms of denial, this type of thinking is designed to keep you sick, not help you to deal with your problem. Do you tell yourself that you are too old, too young, too fat, too successful, too far gone, or too poor to get help? The list is endless. This only contributes to your sickness, not your healing.

Levels of Eating Disorders

To help you determine the extent of your food problem, we would like to discuss the three levels of eating-disordered people. "Food users," the first level, are people who do not eat nutritionally balanced meals. Such people eat fast food for a good majority of their meals or skip them altogether. Their eating is usually irregular with some meals being very big while others are small. Unfortunately, most people in the country fall into this category. Food users are the ones who will "pig out" after a tragic event or for a celebration. While they do overeat on occasion, they are usually able to walk away from food, even ignore it.

The next level is "food abusers," more commonly known as "compulsive overeaters." These are people who binge at least once or twice a week. They think about food a great deal of the time and have unusual relationships with food. They may, for instance, eat one particular food many times during the week or use food repeatedly as a reward or punishment. Food abusers have tried many times to lose weight, even succeeding for a period of time. Their desire for food, however, always seems to win out in the end over their weight-loss efforts. They feel guilty about their eating and are unable to discuss it with others. In the final stages of food abuse, these people begin to experience memory lapses and lose their ability to diet for any length of time. They begin to suffer from persistent remorse about their eating patterns. Their promises or resolutions about losing weight fail. Further, food abusers have experienced some ramifications from their eating. The consequences, for the most part, are much less serious than those that the final level of eating-disordered people experience. This is the "food addict," whose life completely revolves around food.

Food addicts have lost interest in most other areas of their lives, including, in many cases, their personal appearance. Their binges are lengthy, and their obsession with food is overwhelming. They isolate themselves from others and begin to feel as if they have lost their personhood. Their life is filled with fears; their thinking becomes impaired. All dieting ideas become exhausted. Their eating continues in vicious circles, ending in self-hatred. Sexual dysfunction begins, as well as work and money troubles.

Many times food addicts will exhibit grandiose and aggressive behavior toward themselves and others. This is an attempt to cover up their lack of self-esteem by convincing the world of how wonderful they are. Similarly, food addicts will often attempt a geographical escape to distance themselves from their problem. In their mind, moving to a new area will provide the long-sought-after happiness their life is missing.

It is vital to point out that even though you may not be at the critical phase of food addiction, you are not necessarily safe from it. In other words, you are not that bad YET. With perhaps the exception of a very small number of food users, each level is progressive. This means that if you are at the food-abuser level, it is only a matter of time before you reach the chronic phase of food addiction.

Your problem will not magically disappear without getting help. It will only continue to worsen each day. Think about how your eating habits now are different from a few years ago. Do you eat more than ever? Are you less able to diet than you were before? Have you stopped doing certain activities that you used to love so you could have more time to eat? Are you sneaking food when you never did before? Is your guilt about eating getting stronger?

These are all questions you need to ask yourself to discover how your disease has progressed over time. Even if you are at the beginning stages of food abuse, your problem will only get worse unless you do something about it. It is not, however, necessary for you to experience the devastating food-addiction phase before taking action. That is what this book is about. It is an attempt to help you deal with your food problem before it gets to the critical phase. Your problem does not have to get worse.

Throughout this book, we will continue to use the term "food addiction" when referring to both food abusers and food addicts for the sake of simplicity. Considering that the characteristics of the two are similar, except for the degree to which they are experienced, the use of the term is accurate.

Whatever level your eating disorder is at, the fact remains that denial is a powerful mechanism, so powerful that it never truly leaves. There may be times in your recovery from food addiction when you are totally aware of your eating behaviors. Your denial mechanism, however, will still be present in your subconscious, waiting to strike again.

We say this not to scare you, only to warn you of the seriousness of it. Think of denial as the part of yourself that is unable to deal with anything new. When you begin to recover, your denial will try to hamper your efforts. Denial is a protective mechanism that is unable to tell the difference between positive and negative help. It only knows that your present state of mind is threatened. It will work to protect your current situation, no matter how unhealthy and painful it may be. It is for this reason that a discussion about weighing and measuring your food is important.

Weighing and Measuring Your Food

Food addicts have bad eyes when it comes to food. Even after years of weighing and measuring food, many addicts are continually amazed at how inaccurate their perceptions of food can be. Many times they are convinced that the amount of food present is much less than their accepted allotment when sometimes it is twice as much as they needed.

While at first weighing and measuring your food may seem like a prison sentence, there are a few things we would like you to keep in mind. If you do not weigh and measure your food, you will not know exactly how much you are eating. In order to be rigorously honest about your food intake, you must have a system to follow your food plan accurately. Not eating enough food is just as harmful as eating too much. In order to protect yourself from a possible binge or slip off your program, weighing and measuring is necessary.

Think about how many times in the past you have dieted. Where did you have problems? For many food addicts, a lot of it was with their "addict's eyes." They would convince themselves that one cup of vegetables would never be enough to satisfy their hunger, so they never bothered to measure it. Most people, however, don't even know what a cup of vegetables looks like! Do you realize that when you go out to a restaurant, you rarely get even half a cup of vegetables with your meal?

For right now, do not worry about how much food you will be able to eat on the food plan. Instead, understand why weighing and measuring is vital to your recovery. "Eyeballing" your food—using your eyes instead of your cup and scale—is not accurate enough. After a really bad day, half a cup of starch may seem like an eighth of a cup. Also, many addicts report worrying that meals which have satisfied them for years will not be enough to fill them on certain days. It is because of things like this that addicts need to weigh and measure their food.

While these are very important reasons for using a cup and scale, there is a more serious one: when food is not weighed and measured, portion sizes will either increase or decrease. Eventually, this will cause the food addict to stray from the food plan and relapse.

If you eat portions that are too big, the strong denial mechanism will begin to convince you that you really can have three more cups of cereal. This will eventually lead you to believe that you are not really that addicted to food. This will cause you to begin overeating your prime binge foods. And you will be led right back to where you started—desperate and in pain.

If your portions are too small, on the other hand, you will be denying your body the nutrients it needs to function properly. This will set up a deprivation mode of thinking. For example, you will eventually convince yourself that you "deserve" just one cookie for sticking to your "diet" so well. And the cycle of craving will begin all over again. Either way, not weighing and measuring will eventually lead to irrational thoughts that convince you to overeat.

A food addict's mind is only too willing to use any excuse available to overeat. There is no need to contribute to this by eyeballing your food. After all, how difficult do you actually think it is to place a protein on the scale and read the numbers? Keep an open mind about it. At least wait until you read about constructing your personalized food plan before making any final judgments about weighing and measuring your food.

Letting Go

This brings us to another aspect of the denial process. Most food addicts, after using food to comfort themselves for a good portion of their lives, have a difficult time letting go of certain foods. In addition to the physical withdrawal, they will experience an emotional withdrawal. The emotional dependency on food involves a deep-seated belief that the food addict must eat in order to be happy. Food becomes the addict's life—lover, companion, friend, and nurturer.

On the surface this may sound ridiculous, but think about some of your binges. Did you plan them as if they were a social occasion that you had to prepare for? What about Friday or Saturday nights? Were you at home alone with food instead of out with other people? And when you were upset, or even very happy, where did you turn?

In my life, food was used as a substitute for many relationships. My Friday and Saturday nights were planned and prepared for as if they were sacred. Whenever I could, I would get my favorite food—usually chocolate chip ice cream and potato chips—find a romantic movie or book, and eat for the entire evening. Alone in my room, I fantasized that I was the heroine in the movie or book. I just knew my prince would come soon and take me away from my unhappiness.

During these times, food was my lover, friend, and nurturer. It was a visa to the fantasy world I so desperately wanted to be a reality. It was a world where no one knew I was fat. A world where I would be accepted for who I was and, most of all, where I would find that one special someone to love.

For birthdays, anniversaries, holidays, and any other special occasion I could think of, food was used to celebrate. When I was sick or in emotional pain, food was used to make me feel better. Many times I even feigned illness in order to stay home alone and eat. To me, these were my special times when I did something to take care of myself. Some people used Calgon, but I preferred cookies instead.

When it came time to let go of food, I went through a mourning period similar to that of when a loved one dies. Because food was such a big part of my life, I missed it when it was not as prevalent in my daily routine. No longer could I turn to the friend who had seen me through years of pain. Now it was the cause of that pain.

I had to learn to live my life without food being the center of it, and at the time, I thought that was impossible. I could not imagine turning on the television or reading a romance novel without eating something. And what about all those holidays? How would I make it through them? No Christmas cookies or dessert? And on my birthday? How could I be expected to celebrate without a cake? Where would my candles go?

After considering these thoughts, I realized just how big a part of my life food was. What I never understood until now, was that my pain was a direct result of this importance I placed on food. Since I loved eating so much, I never wanted to admit just how much pain it really was causing me.

Can you see how your pain is related to food and your addiction? But more important at this point, do you see how emotionally attached to food you are? Think about your rituals with food. Is there a certain activity you could not imagine doing without eating? What about work? Do you have to eat a certain food there most days? Is it part of your routine? By this, we do not mean a well-balanced breakfast. We are referring to the "bagel wagon" or the "morning jelly doughnut run" that is a part of many office morning routines.

Only One Day at a Time

To recover, you will need to let go of these routines and these foods. While it may be difficult, it is not impossible. Consider the amount of pain and grief that eating these foods has caused you. That should make it easier to think of life without them.

Another way to make letting go of the food easier is to do as Twelve Step recovery groups suggest—take your recovery one day at a time. Only worry about not eating those foods for the next twenty-four hours, just for today.

One of the major psychological reasons I believe that diets failed for me was because I had the next year planned out. I figured out the amount of weight I should lose each week in order to be thin by my designated time. And when I did not meet the unrealistic goals I had set, I got frustrated and overate. By taking it one day at a time, I remove the pressure from myself of staying on my food plan for the rest of my life. As long as I remain abstinent from overeating today, then tomorrow will take care of itself.

It is okay if you do not quite understand the concept of one-day-at-a-time living yet. It takes some people a very long time to fully realize how helpful the notion can be. At this point, just acknowledge that there may be some emotional pain involved with putting down the food. You may feel sad, depressed, angry, even lonely, but it is all right. These feelings are a normal reaction to releasing your addiction.

As you will find out, you are not alone in this. Millions of other people suffer from this disease. It might surprise you to find out that food addiction knows no boundaries. It cuts through all racial, economic, and gender lines. No one is immune to suffering from this affliction, as you will soon discover.

Remember that even though food addicts are each unique in their experiences, they all share certain feelings and characteristics. The emotional pain of releasing food is one of them. For some, the pain of eating is so great that letting go of their food is easy, while others struggle with saying good-bye.

Whatever your experience, realize that your denial will try to fight you in your efforts to recover. This is why it's vital to remain aware of your circumstances.

Still not convinced you've got a problem? Review your food history and your answers to the quiz in chapter 5. Think about your experiences with food. Do whatever it takes to remind yourself of the pain you felt while you were abusing food. Remembrance of this pain is the strongest weapon you have. Use it when the little voice inside of you whispers that you do not have a problem with food, as you munch on a chocolate chip cookie.

8

You're Not Alone

How many times have you thought that you are the only person in the world who does insane things with food? Have you ever deperately wanted to talk with someone about your problem but didn't for fear of being judged? How often have you felt that no one would ever understand the pain you have experienced because of food?

Take heart. This chapter will show you are not alone in your disease. The personal stories in this chapter are taken from surveys and interviews conducted during the writing of this book. Millions of people suffer from the disease of food addiction. The difference between them and you is that you are taking action to deal with your problem. Many food addicts have not even heard of the disease.

Early in my recovery, I was convinced that I didn't need anyone else, and more than that, I certainly didn't need to hear about another person's problems. I was completely close-minded. Then, one day, someone mentioned ordering two of everything, including sodas, when they went to a fast-food restaurant. They did it so the waitress wouldn't know they were going to eat all of the food.

After hearing this, I burst into tears. I could not believe that even one other person in the world had done something I considered to be highly secretive and completely deranged. When the initial shock of it was over, I felt extremely relieved to find someone else who understood me. From that point on, I was able to open up about my eating.

Our hope is that you will find relief in at least one of the personal stories in this chapter. Some of the people are older, some are younger, some have been in recovery for years, and others are only just beginning. Despite their differences, they all have one thing in common—food addiction.

A Long History of Addiction

Chet Sweet of Seattle is a fifty-two-year-old who admits being addicted to sugar (especially fructose), wheat, caffeine, and bulk. He discovered his problem more than twelve years ago when a chiropractor suggested he check for food allergies. After examining his eating patterns, Chet discovered he was severely addicted to several substances. He also found that he could not stop eating them by himself.

"Overeaters Anonymous and the Alcoholics Anonymous Big Book, especially the 'Doctor's Opinion,' helped me get clear that it was physical and truly was just part of a disease of addiction," he said. "Before that I tried a dozen diets and always gained weight back."

After several attempts at abstaining from his trigger foods, Chet had an experience that convinced him of his physical addiction to certain substances. "I went into shock when I added wheat after being withdrawn," he said. "I also had severe headaches from a sip of sugar cola after being withdrawn. While withdrawing I felt hopeless, despair, very tired, cranky and had cravings."

Upon investigation into his family, he discovered a long history of addiction, with his earliest memories being of his grandparents. "My grandmother died of food addiction; she couldn't stop eating though the doctor said she'd have a heart attack. She died at fifty-two," he said. "My grandfather died of alcoholism at forty-six. My father is addicted to religion and work. My mother is codependent and food addicted, and I have two alcoholic uncles, one food-addicted aunt, and a food-addicted nephew."

Today, after changing his eating habits to avoid his addictive substances and through the help of his support group, Chet has lost more than eighty pounds. In addition, he has also stopped bingeing and feeling crazy, is less depressed, and has become more honest both with himself and others. He is currently helping other food addicts to recover. For him, discovering his addictive foods led to a happier, more fulfilling life, free from the craziness of constantly obsessing about food.

Three Who Learned

Marie A., a twenty-three-year-old teacher from Syracuse, New York, also experienced physical symptoms when she began to withdraw from her addictive substances. These symptoms included severe headaches, tiredness, depression, shakiness, low energy levels, and fogginess. Her first lesson about the physical aspects of food addiction came at an Overeaters Anonymous meeting nearly four years ago.

"I had tried many diets—mostly ones that I had made up. I lost weight only once before Overeaters Anonymous and gained it back when people started to notice. Three years and ten months ago I went to Overeaters Anonymous and have been attending meetings on a regular basis," she said.

Unlike Chet, Marie did not have a large amount of weight to lose. "How much you weigh is not important—food addicts can be very 'normal' looking," she points out. "When I add foods I am addicted to into my body, it reacts. It affects the way I think. I've gained energy, enthusiasm, weight loss, and maintenance for three years; clear thinking; and the ability to exercise by discontinuing my use of addictive foods."

Today, Marie is happily married with a daughter and has maintained a twenty-five-pound weight loss. For those still unsure of whether or not they are addicted to food, Marie offers this advice, "If you spend a lot of time thinking about food, what you should eat, what you shouldn't eat, what you are eating, what you're going to eat later, losing weight, gaining weight, then you are probably a food addict."

Another food addict, Frannie, a sixty-one-year-old from Sandston, Virginia, first learned her disease included physical aspects when she realized food was making her ill. "I had cancer and lots of physical problems, bad knees, bad back, high cholesterol, and I was tired all of the time," she said.

Frannie had tried many traditional weight loss methods, as well as some of the more controversial ones, including acupuncture, hypnosis, and fasting. She finally sought help from a food-addiction treatment center. The center provided her with a food plan free of her addictive substances. Frannie discovered that the foods she loved to eat were actually causing her to crave more of the same. Before abstaining from her addictive foods, Frannie's cholesterol was 481. After just two and a half months, it dropped to 220! To date, she has lost forty-one pounds and gained a new incredible life. "I'm a computer operator for AT&T. Before the weight loss I could hardly get myself ready for work because of physical pain," she said. "That's much better now."

While Frannie admits to having a few relapses in her program, she says they have only proved even more to her that she has a disease. "Now I know there's a way to help my disease by eliminating the foods that cause my problem," she said. "I was very depressed before; now I have a feeling of hope and know there is a food plan that will work for me if I work it."

For Denise M. of Bridgeport, Connecticut, knowledge about food addiction came in a very painful way. Her husband died from an obesity-related heart attack at an early age. Despite this tragedy, it took Denise years to discover her own addiction to sugar and flour because of her strong denial mechanism. "The only way I got out of my denial was to hear other people describe my life story," she said.

Before this realization, Denise says she had a very negative attitude, felt sluggish, depressed, and thought about food constantly. In an attempt to deal with her problem, Denise turned to drugs, both legal and illegal, with little success.

"Now, I've stopped all sugar and flour foods and am trying to weigh and measure three meals daily with a snack at night," she said. "I feel more in control of my food intake, I don't have headaches or feel sluggish anymore, and my attitude is much happier. I have higher self-esteem and feel more confident." Today, Denise continues to maintain a healthy weight, though she admits to not always being perfect in her program. Happily remarried to a recovering alcoholic for the past several years, she is evidence that a healthy lifestyle can bring about great change.

One Who Doubts

Jennie H. of New Brunswick, New Jersey, is still trying to come to grips with her food addiction. The twenty-nine-year-old doctoral candidate says she feels more relaxed, calmer, and not as preoccupied with food and food choices when she is abstaining from her addictive substance, sugar. At other times, however, she feels deprived.

She first learned about the physical aspects of food addiction when she was diagnosed with hypoglycemia. Though the initial discussion mostly concerned sugar's effect on her system, it was enough to get her thinking. Like many food addicts, she chose to attend several meetings of Overeaters Anonymous to deal with her problem.

Over the next year, while abstaining from foods high in sugar, Jennie lost sixty pounds and felt wonderful. Her bulimia, which she had struggled with for years, was also in remission during this time. Yet, she remained unconvinced of the addictive nature of sugar. Jennie did not believe her addiction was as serious as a drug addiction. She would admit, however, that sugar had a physical effect on her, evidenced by the headaches and crankiness she experienced during withdrawal.

After her first year, Jennie began to doubt her new way of life. While she knew her past dieting attempts failed, she still struggled with her feelings of deprivation. Eventually, Jennie turned to the sugary foods she wanted. She believes her weight loss and feelings of deprivation led to a major relapse with bulimia.

For the next year and nine months, she alternated between periods of bingeing and purging, resulting in a forty-pound weight gain. Today, Jennie is trying to recapture the degree of recovery she had when she was abstaining from sugar. While she is still not thoroughly convinced of sugar's addictive nature, she admits to being much saner when she removes the substance from her diet. She offers the following advice to fellow food addicts: "Get help somewhere. You're not alone. Whatever you try, realize that you have a disease and that, no matter what, you are not to blame."

Working Again

Paulette D. of Navarree, Ohio, on the other hand, is strong in her conviction about her addictive substances, which she says are sugar, flour, and caffeine. Paulette, a forty-five-year-old nurse, first heard about the physical addiction to food at a program presented during a faculty meeting.

Prior to this, Paulette had gone on restrictive calorie-counting diets of about eight hundred calories a day. "I would lose fifty pounds in four or five months, but the second I went back to normal eating, which meant introducing foods with sugar and flour in them, I would start on a binge cycle of eating and would eventually gain all my weight and more back," she said.

Desperate and full of self-hatred due to many failed dieting attempts, Paulette was unable to work as a nurse for fifteen years. To deal with her problem, she checked herself into a food-addiction treatment center for six weeks. During her withdrawal from sugar and flour, she experienced severe headaches and abdominal cramping. "At the beginning, the concept of abstinence from sugar, flour, and caffeine seemed overwhelming, but by approaching it one day at a time and being willing to just do it, it worked," she said. "For me, it is the only thing that ever worked and it's worth it." More than ten years later, Paulette has maintained a weight loss of about fifty pounds. She had never achieved that prior to giving up sugar, flour, and caffeine. Paulette also has fewer medical problems and much more physical energy. "The greatest progress I've noticed is my freedom of choice to learn to cope with life on life's terms without living in constant fear," she said. "Because of this, I have been able to make decisions and take all kinds of risks, and my life has changed radically for the better. I'm now able to be assertive and voice my needs."

Due to the incredible changes in her life, Paulette was able to return to work a year after treatment. "I now work at a treatment center that deals with alcohol and drug abuse," she said. "This was my heart's desire to work here after I went through treatment myself. It changed my whole life and I wanted to be able to share my experience, strength, and hope with others." Despite the closing of the treatment center, Paulette was able to continue working in her field and eventually find the happiness she had been seeking all of her life. She recently married a fellow recovering food addict and is happier than she's ever been in her life.

How Others Helped

After years of yo-yo dieting attempts, Terri D. from Monroe, Connecticut, learned about her addiction from hearing the experiences of other food addicts. "I tried Weight Watchers and speed diet pills all of my life," she said. "I would get up to 180 to 200 pounds and get divorced, then care enough about myself to get diet pills to lose weight. Before I joined Overeaters Anonymous, I was on my way back up the scale to 160 pounds, but I went there and learned about a lifetime way of eating. I achieved my goal weight of 140 pounds. It was wonderful." To achieve this, Terri gave up eating foods that were addictive for her—sugar, flour, and wheat. She points out that carbohydrates, such as bread, pasta, chocolate, any kind of ice cream, and sugar-free frozen yogurt are especially problematic for her. "I can even binge on abstinent foods," she says. "It scares me all of the addictions I have."

During her withdrawal, Terri experienced light-headedness, irritability, tiredness, and weakness. "I went through the motions of wanting to get up and do something with food, but that wasn't an option anymore, so I needed to do something else like reading, writing, or talking on the telephone," she said.

At the same time, Terri discovered a strong presence of alcoholism and drug addiction in her family. "My father is addicted to food and alcohol too," she said. "He's having a hard time accepting who he is and the role he played in his children's lives. He is looking at who he is and is not liking himself very much. Now he is going to doctor after doctor to achieve physical relief, but it's not working."

Despite the disease she inherited, Terri was able to experience the benefits of abstaining from her addictive substances. "I had more energy than ever. I was able to go to my closet and look good in anything I chose to wear on my body," she said. "My feet didn't ache anymore. I could do any activity I chose to."

Currently, Terri is bouncing back from a devastating relapse during which she gained seventy-five pounds. Though she still has much work to do, she has learned a great deal from the past ten years. She advises other food addicts to "love yourself no matter what. We are all children of God and He loves us just the way we are. Forgive yourself and truly mean it. Know that there is a divine plan for all of us, and we are in heaven on earth each day of our lives. Live this divine love flowing through us every minute and stay focused on the power we have to love and let ourselves love from our hearts every moment." When asked how she is doing today, Terri comments, "I have to say that I am a good person no matter what. I am on my way back down [the scale] very slowly. I have lost fifteen pounds to date."

Like Terri, Julie Bows from Trumbull, Connecticut, also learned about food addiction from Overeaters Anonymous. She points out that she "didn't realize it was an addiction before that. I had tried Physician's Weight Loss Center, Optifast, Slimfast, Weight Watchers, and a slew of book diets. All of them worked in the very short term and failed immediately after. I regained ten pounds each time."

Julie abstained from sugar, which she discovered to be addictive for her. In four and a half months, the fifty-two-year-old human resources manager, who admits to having had a weight problem for more than twenty years, had lost fifty pounds. She also gained an enormous amount of energy.

In Overeaters Anonymous, Julie had found an answer to her

problem and a group of people who understood her. "The camaraderie, understanding, and nonjudgmental atmosphere at Overeaters Anonymous is the only way for me to succeed for a lifetime. People need other people just like them to understand and help," she said. "I'm finally beginning to have self-esteem. I no longer hate myself for my failure to control my addiction."

Sadly, despite Julie's gains, she has recently begun struggling with her food program. During a particularly difficult time in her life when she stopped attending Overeaters Anonymous meetings, Julie turned to food to comfort her and has since been unable to abstain from her addictive foods.

A Difficult Withdrawal

Patti from New Jersey learned about food addiction at an Overeaters Anonymous meeting twelve years ago. Prior to that she had tried many diets, even losing 140 pounds, which she gained back in less than a year. "When I went to my first OA [Overeaters Anonymous] meeting seven years ago, they talked about having a disease and the effects of sugar on your body and mind," she said. "I never truly accepted or understood the withdrawal and addiction concept until I went to treatment."

While in a food-addiction treatment center, Patti learned that she was physically addicted to sugar, fats, dairy products, and most likely white flour. "During my withdrawal, every part of my body hurt—joints, bones, etc. I felt the hair growing on my head, and even my fingernails hurt. I had severe headaches and chills. Someone at the treatment center compared it to chopped meat thawing out. . . . That was accurate," she said. "I also had an intense emotional withdrawal with deep crying."

Although her withdrawal was on the severe side, the benefits she gained after abstaining from her addictive substances was worth the temporary discomfort. "I was able to concentrate and walk much easier. I didn't have chest pains anymore. My heart palpitations stopped, and I didn't gag or choke anymore. I stopped shaking, had more energy, and slept much better," she said. While her physical recovery was very successful,

Patti continued to struggle with the emotional aspects of her addiction. "I went to intensive one-on-one therapy for four years to identify and resolve core issues, but it's very difficult," she said. "I relapsed into my addiction. Now, I'm just starting to see the light."

The forty-three-year-old says that today she feels better emotionally than ever before. Despite gaining weight during her relapse, Patti is back in recovery again and losing weight. She notes that food addiction is a disease, which sometimes includes relapses. But today she knows it is also possible to live a happy, productive life free from her addictive substances and is currently pursuing a new career as a writer.

Success and Loss

Like Patti, twenty-one-year-old Christine from Stratford, Connecticut, struggled to remain in recovery. A gymnastics teacher, Christine had used compulsive exercising to control her weight. She often walked up to twelve miles a day at her most dangerous point.

"My physical addiction to food did not truly begin to take its toll until Christmas of '91," she said. "Before this I was starving myself, bingeing once in a while, then purging by compulsively walking. I didn't believe that I had a problem. Then, I turned away from the compulsive walking and began stuffing my face with anything and everything. I was experiencing drastic mood swings, probably because of my disease. I was put in the hospital and diagnosed with manic depression. I tried to tell everyone there that the problem was food, but no one would hear of it."

During her hospitalization, Christine repeatedly struggled to find an answer to her problem. "I knew food and the underlying issues were destroying me," she said. "In the hospital I gained at least thirty pounds in a month. Then, the doctors popped me some pills and I was released."

Desperate and full of self-loathing, Christine decided to try Nutri/System to lose the weight she had gained. "I felt good about myself [after losing the weight], but I eventually became anorexic. This lasted a few months; then the food began to take its toll again. I ended up in the hospital again, only to find out that no doctor in the world could have helped me. After a few months of compulsive overeating and severe suicidal thoughts, I went to OA." With the help of Overeaters Anonymous, Christine discovered that she suffered from a physical addiction to flour and sugar. "I start shoving my face with every type of food and I just can't stop. I am so addicted to food, especially sugars. Ice cream is deadly for me and so is chocolate. I can never have one. It's two bags and two gallons. Then, I purge and eat even more."

Christine's physical addiction was especially evident to her during her withdrawal period. "I became moody and suffered from severe high and low periods. I experienced night sweats, and I couldn't sleep."

At last contact, Christine had begun losing weight and was working a recovery program. Her program included abstaining from her addictive substances and attending therapy sessions and Overeaters Anonymous meetings. Through this experience Christine had discovered one very important concept: "I don't have to hurt me anymore," she said.

Sadly, after getting her life back on track, Christine suffered from a severe reaction to abruptly stopping her medication for depression and obsessive-compulsive disorder. At the age of twenty-three, Christine experienced a seizure during which she fatally injured herself.

Still Another

Like Christine, Beth from Pittsburgh, Pennsylvania, discovered her physical addiction in a group setting. For Beth, however, it took checking herself into a food-addiction treatment center to become totally convinced. Today, she cites her addictive substances as sugar, flour, caffeine, and fats, and has maintained a one-hundred-pound weight loss for more than five years. "I had failed at all attempts at weight loss until I adopted a food plan which eliminated sugar, flour, caffeine, fats, and uncontrolled volume in conjunction with working a Twelve Step program," she said.

During her initial withdrawal period, Beth suffered from

headaches, depression, nervousness, anxiety, self-pity, and fear. Following that, she was relieved of pain in her joints and feet and experienced an increased energy level. Today, the fifty-three-year-old school bus driver and former school teacher is enjoying a life free from bingeing and obsessing about food. Coupled with a sustained weight loss she never dreamed possible, Beth's life has changed completely.

A Marriage Saved

Now that you have read about some individuals in recovery programs, meet a couple in recovery. Their lives have been changed by abstaining from their addictive substances. Nick, a fifty-one-year-old originally from Brooklyn, New York, and Linda, a forty-six-year-old from Bridgeport, Connecticut, have been married for twenty-five years and have three children.

Throughout their marriage, Nick and Linda repeatedly tried to lose weight, each trying many diet programs. For Nick, it was mostly Weight Watchers and self-starvation diets. Linda turned more toward organized weight-loss methods. Of her most drastic dieting attempts, Linda cites a health-food diet. While on it, she had to drink "black stuff that looked like sewer sludge two times a day without eating," she says. "I was supposed to mix this black powder with tomato juice. It looked exactly like sewer sludge. I used to gag on it. I knew it wouldn't work before I even started. I was just going through the motions hoping it would work." Nick says of Linda's dieting attempt, "Even I couldn't believe she drank that stuff."

Throughout all of their previous weight-loss methods, both Nick and Linda suffered from strong physical cravings for food. "It wasn't so much a feeling of failure as it was of frustration," Nick said. "I'd gone through so many diets and nothing worked. The attraction for food was so overwhelming that I'd give up and start eating everything. Every meal was a binge. I ate until I was stuffed and couldn't move anymore."

In addition to the harm eating was doing to each one of them individually, their family relationships suffered. "I got to the point where I really hated myself. I hated my body. I hated my husband. I hated my children. I hated everything," Linda said. "I used to scream and yell at my children for doing insignificant things like if a clothespin broke in half. I would get so angry over nothing, and I was very resentful and jealous of other people, especially if I thought they had more than I did."

Physically, both were in danger. Linda was at a top weight of 276 pounds with a 24 1/2 dress size. She suffered from three herniated discs and could not walk very far without becoming out of breath. Wearing a size-sixty-two pants at 370 pounds, Nick suffered from chronic headaches and backaches at his heaviest.

The turning point for both came when Nick noticed a co-worker's weight loss. "I asked her how she'd done it," he says. "It was really a case of physical attraction. She'd done what I wanted to, so I was very interested in how she was able to lose the weight." His co-worker introduced him to Overeaters Anonymous, where Nick learned that he had a physical addiction to sugar and flour. "I'd never looked at it as an addiction," he said. "The strong cravings that I'd always had proved it to me. Whenever I smelled fresh-baked bread, I would salivate. As soon as I put down my addictive substances, my sense of smell told me I was addicted to them."

While Nick was experiencing success through his newfound weight-loss method, Linda was struggling with her latest dieting attempt. "I had started Nutri/System when Nick first went to OA. While I was very comfortable with the food plan—it was all prepared for me; I didn't have to do anything except open a package—I was still experiencing food cravings."

At this point, according to Linda, it became a competition. "I kept thinking if he can do it, so can I. We had a diet war going, yet at the same time I saw him changing before my eyes. I kept wondering why he wasn't freaking out like he had before when he dieted. I lived for twenty-three years watching him try to lose the weight, but I knew this was different."

Linda's turning point came when, after dieting for three months, her daughter baked cookies. "When I saw them, I had to have them. I ate a handful of them when Nick went out for a walk. When he came back, I threw them under the couch so he wouldn't see," she said. "Before that, I'd never hidden food from him. I didn't have to because if I wanted something, he usually wanted it too."

Seeing the change in Nick, Linda decided to give abstaining from sugar and flour a try. "I went down kicking and screaming," she said. Linda initially had a hard time abstaining from these substances. "I went through a mourning period over the fact that I couldn't have sugar, and I didn't want to believe that that's what was causing my problems," she said. "Seeing the change in Nick made me realize that I could do it for just one day."

As her days began to add up and her withdrawal period ended, Linda experienced the benefits of abstaining from her addictive substances. "Someone told me to wait twenty days to see if I was really addicted. She told me that if I were, then the urge to eat would leave. When the time was up, it was amazing. The craving to eat sugar and also to eat in between meals was gone."

Since then, Linda's attitude has changed drastically. "I look at sugar now as a poison not only to my body but to my mind as well. It does crazy things to my mind," she said. "It scares me. I was totally out of control when I was eating it. I now consider myself to be like a Sybil. When I eat it, I scream and yell over the smallest things. My husband and my children used to be afraid of me."

So where are Nick and Linda today? Both have lost more than 100 pounds with Nick maintaining a 157-pound weight loss and Linda a 104-pound one for the past two years. Now that she wears a size 16 1/2 dress and he wears size 44 pants, they do things they never imagined possible. "I can actually put on a bathing suit and walk on the beach," Linda says. "I can dance all night. We both bicycle ride, and I don't use the escalator. I can walk up and down stairs. But the most important thing is my tap-dancing class. It's always been a dream that's now coming true."

Both attribute their success entirely to removing their addictive substances from their food plans. Nick eats three moderate meals a day. And Linda has continued to follow the Nutri/System maintenance plan, removing sugar-filled items from it. "A lot of their breakfasts and snacks are loaded with sugar," she said. "And they have little candies that you can buy that I don't eat now that I know. I've never broken my abstinence in two years. This is the longest I've ever done anything."

And their relationship? "We never had anything in common," Linda says. "I like candles. He hates them. He likes TV. I hate it. But now we have something in common: our programs. We go to [Overeaters Anonymous] meetings together four to five times a week. We never went out at night together before. Now we have a lot of fun. We're two entirely different people than we were. Nick said to me the other day that he'd like to marry me again because I am such a different person."

Trying Again

Michele T. from Jamesville, New York, also experienced personality changes when she stopped eating her addictive substances. For her, these include sugar, flour, fried foods, and sugar-free cakes, cookies, and ice cream. The thirty-year-old accountant suffered from severe self-hatred when she first discovered her food addiction.

"I wasn't obese when I came into program," she said. "I had about thirty-five extra pounds on me. It was my head that was obese. I hated myself and how I looked. I thought if the weight would just come off, then my life would be great. Boy, was I wrong. I'd tried everything from liquid diets, diet pills, high carbohydrate-low fat, and Weight Watchers."

Michele was not alone in her weight-loss efforts. "My whole family is addicted to food," she said. "Everyone has a weight problem. We've all been to every weight-loss group over and over again!" Though she has had a few relapses, Michele is now happily in recovery. "I have so much more energy. I don't crave foods or have the desire to overeat," she said. "My weight either drops or consistently stays the same. I am a much calmer person today. I'm happier and less judgmental. I'm more honest about myself and others. I feel better [in my head] about myself and my friendships are truer."

When food addicts begin their recovery, they still have much to learn about this new way of life.

Though she learned a lot upon entering recovery, the most crucial lesson Pat M. from Stratford, Connecticut, experienced happened recently after a devastating relapse. Initially, she lost one hundred pounds by abstaining from her trigger foods, which include sugar and white flour. But, then, the forty-six-year-old administrative assistant "binged on a pure, unadulter-ated sugar item approximately three and one-half weeks ago," she said.

"I was experiencing some heavy-duty feelings in my life about getting older, a hurting financial situation, a precarious situation at work with a most difficult employee to get along with, a hard time in a relationship in my personal life, and sick elderly parents who cause me great concern and worry," she said. "I was out shopping on a Wednesday afternoon with my mom and while at the grocery store, I blatantly picked up an item, tossed it flippantly into my carriage, carted it home, and sat to feed on it several hours later. I hid the item in my house because I don't live alone. I didn't even enjoy eating the item at all because I felt dirty eating it—guilty, shameful, and sneaky."

For Pat, the most ironic part was the results of her binge. "After eating the item, I was devastated mentally. I felt like a failure, a lesser person, a weakling, hopeless. I was able to straighten out my food that night—and each day/night since, but then came the physical pain," she said. "The heartburn began. I thought I was going to vomit; then when I couldn't, I went crazy looking for an antacid. Then the incessant head-ache began. It started at the top of my head, worked its way down both the front and back of my skull, and pounded harder and harder. It lasted at that horrendous level for three full days. The headache was so tremendously severe, it even woke me more than once during the night out of a sound sleep for two consecutive nights."

Unfortunately, the headache was not the only pain Pat suffered. "God was I sick! In the middle of the night, I felt like I was going to puke in bed, and the thought crossed my mind that I would probably die in my sleep, drowning in my own vomit. Then, when I started spitting up bile, I wished I would die to end this misery," she said. "I can't begin to describe how incredibly lethargic the sugar entering my system made me. I was so tremendously logy. I had severe diarrhea. If someone else had told me this happened to them at such a severe level from nothing other than sugar, I don't think I would have believed him or her. However, since I was the deserved recipient of this curse, I am a believer."

So where is Pat today? "It has taken weeks of hard work and dedication to myself and my program to pull out of this 'black hole' I placed myself in. My dignity, self-esteem, physical well-being, and health were tremendously jeopardized by this rebellious act," she said. "Additionally, several weeks later, I have been able to tell by my clothing how severely that binge affected my weight loss. The regaining of some weight is so inconsequential though, compared to the ongoing mental devastation this insane act took as a toll within my life. The bloatedness and weight which I put back on is a precious reminder of the devastating havoc this act caused me. There is no substance on earth worth this type of indignity and pain."

Her advice to others thinking about doing the same thing? "If you're thinking of having even just one of those items, please trust me on this one, it just isn't worth it," she said.

A Lifetime of Addiction

Ed, also from Stratford, Connecticut, can attest to Pat's statement. Overweight since as far back as he can remember, Ed had experienced failed dieting attempts and vicious teasing for years. "In fifth grade, I went clothes shopping in the adult section of Anderson Little and the guy said he couldn't help me, so I had to go to a big and tall men's shop," he said. "I went to the doctor and he gave me diet pills. I was so high from them that I didn't know if I was going home from school for lunch or because it was the end of the day. I stayed back that year."

As Ed grew older, his problems with weight only increased. "I had seasonal friends in junior high and high school. When warm weather came and someone would say 'let's go swimming,' I would find an excuse," he said. "In the summer we fought because I wasn't about to put a bathing suit on."

When Ed got his first job, his thoughts were on food. "I thought 'wow, now I could go out and buy the best food.' I was totally amazed that I could buy food," he said. "Around that time I also discovered alcohol. I bought a lot of drinks so I'd have a lot of friends. The only problem was that the true alcoholics didn't want to eat and I did. So that didn't mix for me."

Finally in 1978, at 427 pounds, Ed decided to try still another diet—a clinic in a nearby town. "It worked. I lost weight," he said. "I drank this liquid chalk, ate my tiny piece of meat and stalk of celery at the end of the day. As I was taking the liquid stuff near the end, I began throwing up because it was so nauseating, but I lost 228 pounds."

At thirty-three years old and slim, Ed says he "had no idea what this world was about." Never having dated before, Ed found girls beginning to notice him. His first relationship was a fantasy, according to him. "The girl wanted free meals, but in my mind it was a date. I bought her a six-thousand-dollar engagement ring one Christmas, but she turned me down. I almost threw the ring out the window I was so upset," he said. "My dog got me through that time. I used to ride around and talk to the dog. It never talked back to me."

After recuperating, Ed asked another girl out to make the first one jealous. "I started out wanting to make the other girl jealous, but the one I asked out turned out to be my wife." After marrying, Ed kept his weight down for a little while before he started to gain it back. "I went from an x-large shirt to a 3x but I didn't want my wife to know, so I bought the same shirt in three different sizes and cut the tags out. When my wife would start asking if I gained weight, I would say 'no, the shirt still fits,'" he said.

Desperate to lose the weight he had gained, Ed tried several more diets until he reached his highest weight ever—520 pounds. He was wearing the largest shirt the big and tall men's shop made, and he had developed sugar diabetes. "My wife was putting on my shoes and socks," he said. "I couldn't even wipe my ass. I had to shower after I went to the bathroom."

He heard about Overeaters Anonymous from the owner of a store where his wife shopped. Through group meetings, he learned about food addiction and made his first attempt at abstaining from his addictive foods. After a relapse where he began eating sugar and flour again, Ed has lost 177 pounds and gained a new life. "I'm learning to accept myself today. I've been my own worst enemy my whole life," he said. "I wore shorts for the first time this summer. I take it one day at a time. I'm in it for the long haul. And my life is very good for today."

Life Becomes Less Manageable

Leona, a forty-six-year-old deli owner from Connecticut had a similar experience. Suffering from food cravings since childhood, Leona says she used to slice a center piece out of a cake her mother had baked. "I was told not to touch it. I would just frost it over so no one knew that I'd eaten any," she said.

As she grew, so did her food intake. "I never really binged so much that I got sick," she said. "I just ate all of the time. It's like I was in a constant state of digestion all the time. I kept food in my car, in my pockets in my pocketbook, everywhere."

Leona's life was also filled with rituals surrounding food. "I would take a Hershey bar and break it in half down the middle and separate the divided sections, then stack them in one pile," she said. "I would eat them as I was working. It was the system I had. With M&Ms, I'd eat all of the brown ones first, then yellow, orange, green, and red for last. The only other way I ate them was to put one of each color in my mouth at the same time."

At over three hundred pounds, Leona found herself limited by her size. "I don't know exactly how far over three hundred pounds I was because my doctor's scale didn't go any higher," she said. "I didn't go to my son's football games because I couldn't walk up the hill when it came time to leave, and I didn't go to college because I wouldn't fit in the seats. The first day I tried, I ended up leaving in a panic."

As Leona's food addiction progressed, her life became less and less manageable. "I had panic attacks. I couldn't even go to the mailbox to get my mail," she said. "I stayed home and ate. I didn't work for seven years. The only places I thought were safe were my car and my house. And the only time I went out was to get food. I would always leave with the pretense of going somewhere else and doing something else, but I only ever went out to eat.

"If I went to the hamburger stand, I would always get a hot dog, a hamburger, two onion rings, and two small Diet Cokes so they wouldn't think I was going to eat the whole thing my-self," she said. "And there was a drugstore I went to where I got my favorite candy bars. I always went to the same places."

Though she could not put a name to her problem, the one thing Leona did know was that she was in pain. "I remember once when I went to the grocery store and bought a big bag of Oreo cookies. As I started eating, I knew something was wrong. I didn't know what it was, but I knew this wasn't nor-mal behavior, so I threw the whole bag of cookies out the car window as I was driving," she said.

That day, she had an appointment with her chiropractor. She told him what had happened. "My chiropractor said he couldn't do any more for me and suggested I go to an Over-eaters Anonymous meeting. I was desperate so I went," she said. "Twelve or thirteen years earlier, I had attended one meet-ing, but I thought they were nuts. But this time it was differ-ent. I knew I belonged. People there were saying things about food, and I felt as if they understood me."

At that meeting, Leona learned about the concept of being physically addicted to certain foods. With the help of another OA member, she began abstaining from her addictive sub-stances. "I sort of believed it was possible to be addicted to food, but I wasn't sure. I was willing to try it," she said.

Even though she suffered from a panic attack during that first meeting, Leona forced herself to stay because she knew it was what she needed. With the help of Overeaters Anonymous and individual counseling, Leona learned to deal with her panic attacks. She has continued to attend meetings while abstaining from her addictive substances.

"During withdrawal, I had bad headaches the first few days and I felt depressed, but I also felt like I was doing something good. I was moving in the right direction," she said. "Once I stopped eating sugar, I didn't crave sugar anymore. Once I stopped eating white flour, I didn't crave white flour anymore. With good therapy, OA, and prescription drugs, I learned to deal with the panic attacks. I had to have all three working together, and I couldn't have done it without my food being in order."

In addition to her food addiction, Leona suffers from drug and alcohol addiction. "A year after I started OA, I got sober," she said. "Alcohol and drugs would calm me down, but food was different. Food is my drug of choice because it's socially acceptable. Nobody ever got arrested for driving under the influence of chocolate."

Despite her initial success with abstaining from her addictive substances, Leona eventually found herself back to where she started. "The first thing I ate [with sugar and flour] was not a problem," she said. "It's not that one thing that got me in trouble. After I ate the first thing, I went right back on my plan for another week until someone asked me if I wanted something. Then I had something else because I got away with the first thing."

Even though she was not following her food plan, Leona continued to attend Overeaters Anonymous meetings. "It was worse after being in recovery because I knew this time," she said. "I knew what I was doing. I didn't know how dear [recovery] was to me until I lost it. I didn't know how miserable I was until I got miserable again."

So, what made the difference for Leona? "I started weighing and measuring my food. I realized that I don't know how much is how much," she said. "I can't judge food like some people can't ride a two-wheel bike. I'm not able to judge how much half a cup of something is for myself."

Since abstaining from her addictive substances once again, Leona's life has changed drastically. "Today, I don't need food to make me happy. I'm not perfect," she said. "The sick part of me wants to believe that someday I'll be able to eat those things again, but not today. I learned that food won't fill the empty parts in my life."

In addition to being free from food cravings, Leona has received many other benefits. These include a seventy-pound weight loss, higher self-esteem, a clearer head, a better thought process, fewer headaches, an improvement in her bad back, less fear about sitting in chairs or going places, the ability to exercise, and the ability to wear sneakers. "I couldn't wear sneakers before," she said. "I couldn't tie my shoes. I had to have slip-on shoes."

The most important lesson Leona has learned? "If I waited until I wanted to work my recovery program, they'd bury me in a piano box," she said. "I don't have to want to do it, I only need to do it. Without recovery, I really believe I'd be worse than dead. I want one person who's suffering to read this and understand that they're not bad people. It's a disease."

Are you that one person? Now that you have read other food addicts' experiences, can you relate them to your own life? Did you read things that you understood and had felt? Of course, you will not relate to everyone in this chapter. If you could empathize with even one person's experience, however, use it as your hope and strength. If they did it, you can too.

And remember, as you are learning how to recover from food addiction, you are not a bad person. And you are not alone anymore. Read on and discover your trigger foods. Recovery from food addiction can be yours too. You are truly not alone.

9

Finding Your Trigger Foods

In this chapter, you will take concrete steps toward developing a personalized food plan. It is time for you to put into action all that you have learned so far. We have been asking you to do various exercises that were designed to help you find those foods most dangerous for you. If you have completed these exercises, you may already be aware of the most glaring of your problem foods. This chapter will help you to discover other foods that cause you difficulties. If you have not done the exercises in chapter 5, it may be a good idea to go back and complete them (see pages 53–55, 57, 58).

What Are Trigger Foods?

Before we go on, it is necessary to define "trigger foods." Trigger foods are those foods that, when you eat them, cause you to continue eating, most likely bingeing. You may or may not eat these foods on a regular basis. It doesn't matter how many times you eat a trigger food—what matters is what the food does to you once it is in your system.

> Potato chips were one of my biggest trigger foods, yet I hardly ever ate them. Instead, I ate popcorn every day. I rationalized in my mind that popcorn was a better "diet food" than the potato chips I loved so much.
>
> Whenever I ate potato chips, I never had just one. Yes, but many non-food addicted people cannot eat just one chip

either, you are arguing, right? The difference is, for me one potato chip led to eating the entire bag and, at the very least, a half gallon of chocolate chip ice cream. Most times, I ate much more than the two items mentioned and made myself extremely sick.

Think of an alcoholic who drinks only on weekends. Because the drinking is not regular, alcoholics are able to convince themselves that they do not have a problem. Yet, each weekend is spent either passed out or drinking everything in sight. While it is clear to you that this person has a drinking problem, it may not be so obvious with your food addiction. As we have told you, food is not considered as harmful as alcohol, even though for some people it is just as dangerous.

Are there certain foods that you reserve for special occasions or weekends? When you eat them, do you almost always eat more and more and more? Even, if after eating them, you turn to what you consider healthy foods, your answer should still be yes. As you now know, all so-called healthy foods are not necessarily good for you.

Discovering Your Trigger Foods

To discover your trigger foods, first take out your food history and begin to look for patterns. If you have thoroughly and accurately written down your binges, some of your trigger foods will be glaringly obvious. Others you will have to search for. For now, just notice the foods you continually turn to when you binge. Is it only one particular food or are there many foods of one type? For example, do you always eat foods high in sugar or fats? flour? wheat? Think about the texture of these foods. Are they usually crunchy? sweet? gooey? soft?

What about the condiments you eat with the foods? Do you use a lot of butter or even margarine? oil? mayonnaise? ketchup? mustard? chocolate sauce? nuts? syrup? Even if you are convinced that what you eat is a completely healthy food, if you binge on it, write it down. We will show you later how so-called healthy foods can be dangerous triggers for many people. Just make your list; worry about analyzing it later.

If you did not complete a food history and are not willing to, then think about your food patterns. It would be best to consider the past week. Think about a different time period, however, if during the previous week you have been trying some new crash diet or other method of weight loss that has drastically altered your eating patterns. Think about the foods you have eaten. Also, look for definite patterns in the times and amounts of food.

Be warned that relying solely on your memory will not be nearly as effective as a written record of your eating history. Also keep in mind that you will get out of this book exactly the amount of effort you are willing to put forth. You cannot expect a strong recovery if you are not willing to work for it. As always, the choice is yours.

Making a List

After you have reviewed your past and have identified your eating patterns, write them all down on a separate sheet of paper. It may even be helpful to title the paper "My Trigger Foods." You will use this list in chapter 11 when you create your personalized food plan.

When making this list, include foods that you have a strong emotional attachment to. You can recognize these by your own feelings. If, for example, you are hesitant, even angry, about including a certain food on your list, it is probably a trigger food for you. If you feel excited about eating certain foods each day, or are frightened to be in the same room with any, include them on your list.

Your emotional response to a food is tied to the denial mechanism you read about earlier. A food addict's denial can be extremely powerful, and some of your trigger foods may be deeply buried beneath a mound of denial. Examining your feelings about certain foods is a very effective way of amassing a complete list of your trigger foods. We usually only have strong feelings—either negative or positive—about those things we care about most. In the case of food, those things you care about most are the ones that may very well destroy you. Unless, of course, you are able to uncover them.

Complete a preliminary list of your most obvious trigger foods. Then ask yourself some questions that may reveal problem foods you may be forgetting. Start with naming foods from your childhood that you considered to represent the ultimate reward, expression of love, feeling of safety, or incredible taste. These foods do not have to be ones you ate on a regular basis. They can be ones you frequently fantasized about or enjoyed excessively.

> If you are, as I am, unable to remember your childhood, it may be helpful to question your parents or other members of your family about this. Only do this if you feel comfortable. I discovered a problem food of mine from childhood quite by accident. My parents would frequently tell me that I needed a vanilla ice-cream cone to keep me from crying during the half-hour trip to my grandmother's house. I was five years old at the time.
>
> While I have absolutely no memory of this experience, I also have no doubt about its truth. Hearing about it helped me to see more clearly just how much of a problem food ice cream is for me even in adulthood. It is sort of like being a detective when trying to identify trigger foods. One clue will lead to several others, which will in turn provide a complete and thorough listing of problem foods.
>
> The difficulty I had with discovering my trigger foods was due to my unquestioning acceptance of them for years. The story I told you about was commonly and quite frequently brought up throughout my childhood and teenage years. I considered it to simply be a part of my history. I never even questioned it or considered that it might contain valuable information about my trigger foods. I only viewed it as one of those cute little stories all parents tell others.

Your past probably contains similar incidents. The easiest way to deal with such occurrences is to go in with a questioning attitude. Question everything. Do not drive yourself crazy or take this to extremes, but seriously question those things that you are absolutely positive have nothing to do with food. In many cases, you will be surprised at how much of your past involves food.

Remember, you have to break through your denial in order to find your trigger foods. You must outsmart the mechanism that works to keep your life in a status quo mode. Is that what you really want, for things to continue as they have been with food? Of course not, or you would not have read this far. Just keep questioning your relationship and experiences with food, and you will find your triggers.

If you do decide to approach your family members about your childhood experiences with food, know that uncomfortable feelings for both parties may arise. Discussing the past may not prove painful for some food addicts' families. For others, however, recalling the past accurately will be nearly impossible due to the amount of denial present. If you are determined to discuss the matter, bring it up in a nonthreatening, matter-of-fact manner to avoid possible confrontations.

Keep in mind that it is not necessary to do this. Your recovery does not depend on extracting some hidden bit of information from your family members. It may, in some cases, be helpful, but it is by no means vital. The only person your recovery depends on is you. No one else can sabotage your recovery, unless you let them.

After examining your childhood for possible trigger foods, take a look at your teenage years. These years may be the most significant indicators of your eating behavior. During adolescence, you were more capable and had greater opportunities to make your own food decisions. This is unlike the helplessness of being told what to eat in childhood. As a teenager, you began to eat meals and snacks independent of your parents' watchful eyes, making this a good indicator of your developing eating patterns.

When you examine this period in your life, look for emerging similarities. Is there one type of food you consistently ate whenever you were not with your parents or another family member? Was there some kind of food that made you feel especially loved, safe, and cared for? Or, did you think that eating a certain food made you "cool"?

By asking myself these questions, I realized that in my early teenage years I went around sucking on sugary lollipops for an entire summer. I thought it made me look very cool. I had seen one of the most popular girls in school with one, and I wanted to be exactly like her. I developed a two-pop-a-day habit. Prior to this, I had lost nearly one hundred pounds and was the thinnest I had ever been. After that summer, I gained just about all of the weight back. The amount of concentrated sugar I was eating, coupled with my cravings for more, took its toll on my waistline.

I also discovered that a chocolate pudding dessert my sister made represented holiday celebrations for me. I would begin to get excited at least two weeks before I knew I was going to be able to eat it. All through the meal I anticipated how wonderful the dessert would taste. I always made sure to hide some for later. Many times I coerced my sister into making a special helping just for our family in case everyone ate all of the other one.

Of course, there were the usual holiday cookies and even ice-cream cake that I began eating several weeks before the celebration. Each holiday was a license to eat everything in sight without feeling guilty or ashamed. It was, after all, a holiday, so how could I be expected to stick to a diet?

Also, for me, getting my license and a job was a special time. It meant that I had the money and the transportation to eat whatever I wanted whenever I could. Many times after working at night, I would tell my parents I was going out with co-workers to the movies. I actually went to a fast-food restaurant to sit in the parking lot and eat. I felt safe in the darkness of my car. I was sure no one could see me.

As I stuffed down two quarter-pound cheeseburgers, two large fries, two large diet sodas, and an apple pie, I watched young couples together. All the while, I wondered why no one loved me. What was wrong with me that I couldn't find a boyfriend or even a friend? Despite the pain of loneliness, these nights represented to me the time I took just for myself. I had always heard and read about women needing personal time, so this was how I took mine. What I did not know then was that my personal time was killing me.

As you look for trigger foods in your adult life, think about the meal choices you make. Do you always cook the same special meal when you want to impress company? What about your children? Do you limit them or reserve a certain food for special occasions? If so, this food is likely a trigger for you. Or, do you have a favorite food that you give as gifts to friends or family?

> In college, as you read earlier, I made batches of chocolate chip cookies, many times passing them out to people who I wanted to be my friends. Mostly, I baked them for a man I was trying to impress. I wanted him to know what a good cook I was so he would want to marry me. Because of this, I continually supplied him with dozens of chocolate chip cookies, even cooking many full meals for him. I believed this would make him love me.

Have you used food in a similar way? If so, examine the types of food you have chosen. In most cases, food addicts give others the same kind of food they enjoy eating—those items that carry emotional connotations with them. If your parents or grandparents consistently fed you a certain food that you began to associate with love or nurturing, you will most likely follow the same pattern. This may be on an unconscious level, however. Even if you are convinced that the foods you eat most are free of sugar, flour, fats, or caffeine, include them in your list anyway.

> I was entirely certain that the popcorn I loved to eat daily did not contain any of the substances I knew to be addictive. Since there was no sugar or flour in popcorn, then why did I binge regularly on it? What I did not take into consideration was that I soaked it in butter or bought the butter-flavored type. Both of

these contained large amounts of oil. Even the plain micro-wavable popcorn had oil in it. And, as you already know, fats are highly addictive.

These are the types of connections you will need to notice. The best rule to follow when making your list is this: if you eat it a lot and look forward to it even more, include it. Do not worry about whether you will have to stop eating the foods you list. Simply include it, and later on, we will examine whether or not it is a major trigger food. For now, just make the list.

Trigger Foods Quiz

The following questions may help uncover some more of your trigger foods.

1. What foods do you overeat on a regular basis?
2. Of these foods, do most contain one substance, such as sugar, flour, fats, or caffeine? If so, include that in your list.
3. After eating these foods, do you usually eat other foods that contain the same substance? For example, eating chocolate then cookies—both have sugar.
4. Name the foods that you lose control over.
5. List the foods you eat only when you are alone.
6. When you are emotionally upset or physically sick, what foods do you eat to make you feel better?
7. What types of foods do you have hidden around the house?
8. After dieting or starving yourself, what is the food you usually reach for first?
9. Is there any food you lie about eating? If so, name it.
10. What foods do you constantly think about eating? Include those you think about but do not actually eat.
11. When you think of dieting, what are the foods you feel sad about not being able to eat anymore?

12. Over the years, what foods have you drastically increased your intake of on a consistent basis?

13. Does your personality change when you eat certain foods? If so, include these foods on your list.

14. Are there certain foods, even if only for special occasions, that you get excited thinking about eating or preparing?

15. What foods do you make absolutely sure that you never run out of?

16. If you black out or do not remember when you eat a certain food, include it on your list.

17. Can you think of a food that you would rather die than go without eating?

18. If you were stranded on a deserted island and could have any food you wanted with you, what would you choose?

19. When you go out for a meal, is there a certain food you always eat or think about ordering?

20. What foods would you spend your last dollar on?

These questions are only one method of getting you to think about your trigger foods. If you have written a food history and answered the questions, then you have a pretty good idea of what your trigger foods are. You may discover additional ones as you read. For now, we will use the foods you have listed to discover what substances you are most addicted to.

Reading Food Labels

The next exercise may be difficult because of the way food manufacturers often disguise the presence of sugar and other substances by using fancy names. There are ways, however, to identify the substances in your binge foods.

First, we will start with a basic lesson about sugar. As we've already discussed, sugar is in nearly every packaged food available today. The tricky part is that it is often called a different name. To date, we have found twenty-one different names for sugar! Medical experts from the University of California,

Berkeley, point out, "Even when a label claims 'sugar free' it still can contain some type of caloric sweetener, and one form is no more nutritious than another."[1]

Here are the other names for sugar that are used today[2]:

barley malt	honey
brown sugar	invert sugar
cane sugar	lactose
corn sweetener	maltose
corn syrup	mannitol
dextrose	maple syrup
fructose	sorghum
glucose	sorbitol
grape sugar	sucrose
grape sweetener	high fructose corn syrup

Using this list, examine the contents of the foods you binge on most. Do many of them contain one or more of these ingredients? Even if you are positive that your favorite binge food does not contain sugar, check the label. You may be surprised. It is also important to remember that foods marked "low fat" usually contain some form of sugar. The reason for this is to make up for the lack of taste once fat is removed.

> Several years ago when grocery shopping, I noticed that my favorite dressing also came in a low-fat version. I decided that it could not hurt to decrease my fat intake, so I examined the label. I found that the first or second item on the list of ingredients for the low-fat version was a form of sugar! I found it completely absurd that I was able to eat the "regular" version, which contained absolutely no sugar, but not the low-fat one.

Examining the labels of your binge foods will help you find the substances you are addicted to. Next, we will list some items that contain sugar, which you may believe are "diet" foods or foods that couldn't possibly be addictive.

Read Your Cereal Box

As discussed, many products labeled "nonfat" or "light" contain large amounts of sugar. Did you know, for example, that most boxed cold cereals, and some hot ones, are loaded with sugar? This includes those advertised as being low in sugar. I am certain you realize that a lot of popular cereals contain sugar; what you may not know is that so-called healthy cereals have, in some cases, just as much sugar.

Take Frosted Flakes, for example. Most people know that the flakes are frosted with sugar. Do you realize that Special K, which many believe to be a diet food, is also very high in sugar? This is true of many granola or natural cereals, as well. Muselix, thought to be a healthy cereal, contains brown sugar, while Raisin Bran also lists sugar in its list of ingredients.

Remember, brown sugar is still sugar and just as dangerous as refined sugar for a food addict. Many health-food products attempt to portray brown sugar as being safer and more natural to eat. For food addicts with a sugar addiction, there is no such thing as "safe" sugar.

Of those other cereals that promise no sugar, many are sweetened with fruit juice. Fruit juice in such a concentrated form contains a great deal of natural sugar. This can be a problem for many food addicts. More details about the difference between natural and processed sugar will be discussed in chapter 11. Additionally, many cereals, both hot and cold, attempt to disguise the presence of sugar by including "honey" in the list of ingredients. As you have already learned, honey is another name for sugar. Beware of anything containing honey if you have a problem with sugar.

Similarly, some cereals will use labels such as sucrose, fructose, or maltose to disguise the presence of sugar in their products. A good rule of thumb is to remember that anything ending in "ose" means sugar. These ingredients will cause food addicts with sugar sensitivities to crave more sugar.

So, what cereals are safe to eat for a food addict? Grapenuts, Shredded Wheat, and Kashi are all free of sugar and fruit juice, as well as nearly all of the Grainfield cereals.

Take a look at the list of ingredients on the boxes of cereals you love so much. Do they contain any of the ingredients listed in this chapter? Are they fruit juice sweetened? If so, think about the amount of cereal you eat. Have you ever binged on cereal?

> I went through a phase in my life during high school when I ate bowl after bowl of Frosted Flakes. I told myself that cereal could not possibly be bad for me to eat because there was not any chocolate or whipped cream in it. For some people, who are not addicted to sugar, Frosted Flakes can be an acceptable meal. For me, however, it led to devastating binge after binge.

Check the Label

Besides cereal, you must be careful of many other breakfast foods if you are addicted to sugar. You know that doughnuts and syrup contain large amounts of sugar. But did you know that frozen waffles and pancakes, especially those with a fruit flavoring, have sugar? Check the list of ingredients! Some yogurts contain sugar, as well as concentrated fruit juice. Even if the label says 100 percent fruit juice, the concentration of the fruit juice is extremely high in order to provide a pleasant taste. This often triggers cravings in food addicts.

If you have an addiction to sugar, you must be equally cautious at lunch- and dinnertimes. Again, items that you would not expect to contain sugar do. Brown rice is okay, right? That depends. Many boxed brown rice dishes include sugar in the flavoring. This is also the case with most boxed side dishes, such as scalloped and mashed potatoes, pasta mixes, tuna and hamburger flavorings, and taco mixtures.

Some meats are a danger too. Kielbasa, some other sausages, most hot dogs, many lunch meats, ready-to-eat barbecued chicken and ribs, and just about all brands of ham contain sugar. Only a few brands of hot dogs do not contain sugar, including Hebrew National and Nathan's. Only one type of ham is free of the substance. Sorry, I did not get the brand name.

Also be wary of the condiments and spices you use in your

cooking. Most tomato sauces contain sugar, and just about all international flavorings include the substance. Aunt Millie's Traditional Meatless Sauce, Francesco Rinaldi Low Salt, Classico Traditional, Victoria's Tomato and Basil, Rao's Marinara, and Stop & Shop Meatless tomato sauces are the only ones I know of that do not contain sugar. While most spices, on the other hand, are safe, a few do contain sugar. Natural vanilla flavoring, not imitation, most lemon and pepper flavorings, and just about all taco seasoning mixtures include sugar.

Liquid condiments can also be dangerous for food addicts. Almost all ketchups, soy sauces, steak sauces, and barbecue sauces contain sugar, as do some mayonnaises and even a few mustards. Kikkoman soy sauce and most plain mustards, such as Guldens and French's, are among the safest. They are also among the best tasting condiments for food addicts.

Now, let us examine salad dressings. We have already touched on how manufacturers use sugar to improve the taste of dressings labeled low fat. Did you know that different flavors of the same brand contain sugar, while others do not. Many regular, not low-fat, Marie's dressings are free from sugar. These include such delicious flavors as Italian garlic, blue cheese, sour cream and onion, ranch, and caesar. Poppy seed and honey dressing, however, contains sugar.

Sugar-Free Desserts

At first glance, sugar-free chocolate, ice cream, cakes, and cookies may seem the most likely substitute for people with sugar addictions. This is not the case. The reasons for this are twofold. First, as we mentioned earlier, food addiction is a complex disease. This includes an emotional element that must be discussed regarding sugar-free sweets.

For those addicted to flour, sugar-free desserts are particularly dangerous. Even if one of your trigger foods appears to be "innocent" of your addictive substances, pay attention to the following information.

When you begin to develop your personal food plan, you will need to consider many things in order to avoid your trigger foods. For example, in the case of chocolate, your physical addiction to sugar is most likely the primary reason you binge.

Some food addicts also binge because they believe they can find safety, nurturing, and comfort in their binge items. If you always turned to chocolate whenever you were upset, eating chocolate again, even the sugar-free variety, may cause you to binge. Eating it could trigger a binge that involves even more dangerous foods, including those that actually contain sugar. Additionally, turning to chocolate when you are upset will not help you to develop healthy emotional coping skills.

The texture of some foods may pose a problem for many food addicts, as well. Foods that are crunchy, creamy, smooth, or excessively soft often trigger binges. For example, many food addicts can eat an acceptable amount of baked potato. Mashed potatoes or french fries, however, result in negative consequences, such as a binge. The texture of soft, creamy mashed potatoes and the crunchiness of long, thin french fries often triggers a negative response in many food addicts. This is because the feeling of actually chewing is intensely enjoyable.

The expectations from food that many addicts hold can also be extremely dangerous. Addicts, especially when they are very happy or unusually sad, turn to food as a way of comforting themselves. Since food has soothed them most of their lives, it is the first place most addicts look to "stabilize" uncomfortable feelings, even if they are positive emotions. Addicts are unfamiliar with experiencing their emotions. The taste of their favorite foods and bingeing on them represents the safety and comfort they believe is needed to feel better.

Either way, eating sweets, even those without sugar, can quickly lead an addict to the "real thing." This is due to the progressive nature of the disease. Food addiction, similar to alcoholism, will only worsen over time if it is left untreated. As evidence of this, consider your past eating experiences. Have they not gotten worse over time?

The second reason to be wary of sugar-free sweets is that the taste of them may cause a binge. As you have read, medical studies have proved that sweet-tasting foods cause those with a preference for them to overeat once introduced into their systems. Once food addicts taste the intense sweetness of the sugar-free items, it will most likely trigger a binge. This may result in eating the foods that are so dangerous to their systems.

Addiction to Flour

There are several things you must think about to determine if flour is a trigger food for you. Does your food history reveal that you eat excessively large amounts of bread, bagels, and batter-dipped items? Waffles, pancakes, french toast, and cereals also contain flour.

> When I first thought about the possibility that I was addicted to flour, I was positive that it could not be so. Sure, I ate a lot of bread, but there were long periods of time when I stayed completely away from it. I was positive it could not be a problem for me. What I failed to realize is that I had developed a habit of eating fried tortillas at least three or four times a week. I also ate tacos on a regular basis. It never occurred to me that these items had flour in them.

Examining Your Eating History

When reading the ingredients on a package, look for similar ingredients in foods you continually binge on. Chances are they contain one or more of the addictive substances mentioned in this book.

What if you binge on meat? There is certainly no sugar or flour in that. You are right, unless of course it is breaded or cooked in a sugary sauce. If neither of these things is true, then you may have a problem with fat. Do you eat a lot of sausages, bacon, butter, fried foods, kielbasa, or ham? These foods contain large amounts of fat, which can also be a highly addictive substance for many food addicts.

All of these things are important to keep in mind when looking at your trigger foods. The most important thing to remember, however, is to be rigorously honest when attempting to discover your problem items. It may be tempting to rationalize

why certain foods are not harmful to you. But doing so will
only hurt yourself.

> If you are not painfully honest about those foods that cause
> you so much trouble, your life will not change. If you are like
> me, you have already tried every diet conceivable with disas-
> trous results. Take the time to discover your trigger foods. By
> doing this, you are moving a step closer to having the kind of
> life you have always dreamed of—free from obsessing about
> food.

The exercises in this chapter help you find your addictive
foods—and give you tools for a better life. Whether or not you
follow this program, completing these exercises will make you
much wiser about your eating patterns. You will know exactly
when you are most vulnerable to overeating, which may help
prevent future incidents.

Either way, knowledge about your trigger foods is the most
effective weapon you have against your food addiction. Again,
awareness is the key to a healthier, happier life free from the pain
of food addiction. You have a choice. You can either continue to
read on or do nothing and remain in pain. But before you decide, remember that the disease of food addiction is progressive
in nature. This means that your pain will only worsen. Your life
will not improve unless you take steps to make it better.

There may be periods in your life where you honestly believe
you have your addiction under control. You want to believe
that you are cured and that you will never overeat again. Unless
you take concrete action toward recovering, you will only go
back to the pain you have always known.

The choice is yours. Only you can decide if the effort is
worth the reward.

10

Abstaining: Today Is Monday

After reading about other food addicts and identifying your trigger foods, you may be convinced that you have a problem. And you might even be ready to start doing something about it. You may be planning to skip ahead to the chapter about developing your food plan. That way you can begin working your program on Monday, right? Read this chapter first. The fact that the mere thought of waiting until Monday entered your mind indicates how much you need this chapter. What is wrong with waiting until Monday, you ask? It seems like a logical starting point, doesn't it?

Sure, at first glance, Monday does seem to be the organized way of beginning your new program of recovery from food addiction. But think about how much food you can eat before Monday comes. And more important, all of the excuses you can concoct before you actually begin. These things may change your mind. Remember the man mentioned earlier who died the night before he was due to be admitted to a food-addiction hospital? How many Mondays do you think he waited before making the decision?

The point is this: you may not have too many more days left, never mind Mondays, if you do not take action right now. Further procrastination on this matter will only lessen your chances of actually recovering from your disease. The longer you wait, the harder it becomes to actually begin.

We are sure you are feeling quite overwhelmed, even some-what depressed at the idea of beginning a food plan. These feelings are quite natural. Many food addicts report being ter-rified of actually starting a program that may truly work for them. That is the funny thing about most human beings—we are just as afraid of success as we are of failure.

> Before beginning my food plan and hearing about the concept of abstaining from addictive foods, I was convinced that it was not possible to live without sugar and flour. What was left, I asked myself? Was I doomed to a life of tasteless vegetables? Could someone really exist without sugar? Wasn't that bad for a person?
>
> After I started following my current food plan, I was shocked at how much food I could actually eat and still lose weight. I was even more surprised at how tasty the food turned out to be. My ability to stay on the food plan also had a strong impact on me. I could not believe that I was actually able to eat three meals a day with a snack at night and not be hungry. It had never been like that for me before. It can be like that for you too.

Perhaps the most effective way of dealing with your fears is to ignore them. Follow your plans despite your fears. As simplis-tic as this sounds, it is not as easily done. It takes a concerted effort to force fear thoughts out of your mind.

Positive Affirmations

One of the easiest ways you can rid your head of fear thoughts is to consistently provide yourself with productive, positive messages. For example, if you constantly think about how scary failure would be, tell yourself you are confident and successful. If, on the other hand, you feel horribly anxious whenever you fantasize future success, then tell yourself that you are enjoying your life now. Keep reminding yourself that you are reaping the benefits of the hard work you have done to this point.

Repeating these positive thoughts, called affirmations, to

yourself on a regular basis will help to diminish your fears. If you are willing to take the time to use them, affirmations can be a very important part of your recovery. Some medical experts even advocate using affirmations in conjunction with traditional treatment to increase the speed and ease of recovery.

The first step in using affirmations is to think about how you would like your life to be. Next, put your thoughts in a sentence and repeat it to yourself on a consistent basis. When inventing your sentence, make sure it is in the present tense. Say, "I am attractive" instead of, "I am becoming attractive," as using the future tense will keep your heart's desire just beyond your reach.

Also, use only positive affirmations. Tell yourself that you are beautiful; do not say, "I am not ugly," because your subconscious is unable to understand the word "not." If you say, "I am not ugly," your subconscious will hear "ugly" more than any other word. You certainly don't want that, do you?

Affirmations are a way to talk yourself out of being afraid and into being the confident, healthy person you desire. Here's how it works: If you continually walk around thinking about how afraid you are, for instance, begin thinking instead that you are confident. If you see yourself as a failure, start using affirmations to tell yourself how successful you are.

By using affirmations, you will become more and more comfortable with the ideas you continually express. When you first begin using affirmations, you may experience some internal resistance in the form of negative thoughts. Because your subconscious is not familiar with positive messages, it will attempt to counteract them with negative thoughts. If you are patient and persistent, however, you will triumph. Once your mind becomes accustomed to the nurturing messages, your life will begin to change.

Does this sound like a lot of work to you? Well, think about this—you already use affirmations in your life, though they may not be positive ones. How many times have you told yourself how fat, ugly, or disgusting you are? Or have you ever informed yourself about all of your shortcomings? Do you do this on a

regular basis? How many times during the day do you find
something to criticize about yourself? Are your clothes too
tight? Is your hair a mess? Is your nose too big or are your eyes
too far apart? Telling yourself these things regularly shows you
are using affirmations. By using negative affirmations, you are
making the very things you want to change about yourself
worse. Whenever a negative thought enters your mind, find its
positive equivalent. It's easy. Repeat it over and over again until
it becomes a reality in your life. By continually reinforcing the
positive messages in your mind, you are laying the foundation
for these things to actually happen.

Early in my recovery, my counselor suggested I use the affirmation "I am likable, lovable, and capable" whenever I thought
otherwise. After using it for a few months, I began to see considerable results. I no longer criticized myself as harshly as I
once did. I began to see a few of my positive traits and even
started to like myself.

One of the most powerful examples of how my affirmations
worked came during a weekend trip to Los Angeles. I had flown
to California to visit a friend, and we had decided to travel to
L.A. for the weekend. My friend, an airline employee, had to fly
on standby while I had a reservation. Upon boarding the plane,
I learned that my friend would not be able to join me on the
flight and would have to find another one.

After landing in L.A. and collecting my baggage, I was overcome with fear, convinced that I was going to be stranded and
desolate in the airport. Negative, critical thoughts filled my
mind as I began to panic. I felt inadequate and unable to take
care of myself.

Then, all of a sudden, a feeling of calmness washed over me
as a thought popped into my mind. I was reminded that I was
capable. I knew then that I could handle whatever happened. All
those months of using my affirmation had worked. While I was
relieved to find my friend a few minutes later, I was even happier
to have felt so confident. Even more, I was grateful for the valuable lesson learned about the effectiveness of affirmations.

Visualization—Another Helpful Tool

Another very useful tool in dealing with fear is visualization, the process of mentally picturing your desired outcome. The theory here is that if you can actually see yourself achieving your goals, your subconscious will work to make them a reality. Some medical experts have used this concept to heal cancer patients with remarkable results.

So, where do you begin? Find a quiet spot and relax. If it will help you concentrate, put on some soft music. Be careful not to choose anything that will require your attention. Make sure to turn off the television. Choose a comfortable position; many people prefer to lie down. Then, think about what you would like your life to be like. Where will you live? What kind of job will you have? How will you look? What will your relationship with food be? Picture the kind of clothes you will be wearing and how you will feel. Will you be proud of yourself? confident? happy? excited? fulfilled? grateful? Whatever it is, visualize yourself at that point in your life.

Be careful not to be unrealistic in your images. For example, picturing yourself as Suzanne Somers is not helpful. This will only cause your subconscious to become frustrated and angry because it is unable to achieve your desired results. Picturing yourself as another person causes you to destroy your own self-worth and leads to resentment and frustration.

The best way to approach a visualization exercise is to imagine yourself at your peak—the best possible person you can be—on a consistent basis. Do not think of all the things you believe are wrong with you. Instead, think of developing your most favorite character traits into the best person you can be. If you are like most food addicts, one of the top priorities in your life is to have a thin body. What does your slim body look like? Picture the clothes you would wear. Are they items you could not possibly fit into now? What size are they? Are you wearing colors that you would not dream of wearing in your present condition?

Once you have a clear picture of yourself and how you want to be, use this image on a daily basis. It will take practice. The most effective time is either right before bedtime or immediately after waking up in the morning. It does not have to take a long time. A minute or two of seeing yourself as you want to be is all that's needed, provided you are persistent and reasonable in your visualizations.

> For me, visualization, though I did not call it that then, literally saved my life. For years when I was eating and feeling hopeless about ever leading a normal life, I carried with me a faint image of myself as thin and happy. I could see myself dressed up and running in a big city with an enormous smile on my face. And whenever I had overeaten or failed at another dieting attempt, that image would always come into my mind.
>
> It was not something I purposely thought of, yet it always seemed to appear at my darkest moments, the ones when I was contemplating suicide. I wanted to escape the pain so desperately that, at the time, suicide seemed like the only way out. I believed I had tried everything else. But this image of myself kept offering me the little thread of hope I needed to continue living. Whenever I saw it, I was continually amazed at how happy I seemed to be. My smile was huge and my face glowed with pride and gratitude for the way my life was.
>
> There were many times that I did not believe I could actually be like this. But there was also this tiny voice inside telling me that I would not always be so miserable and unhappy. Today, I believe that the image I had of myself, along with that voice, saved my life many times. During my most painful moments, I desperately clung to the hope that someday I really would be thin. Since I did not want to miss that, I never actually attempted to end my life.
>
> That image did come true in my life. I am at a normal weight. And I do have a glow about me, one that comes from the pride and gratitude of making my life better, once I was shown the way. I still do not understand the part of the image about being dressed up or running through a big city. I have not gotten there yet. But, if it is as wonderful as the first half of my visualization, I cannot wait!

Using positive affirmations and visualizations will help you lessen any fear you may have about beginning this program. And these exercises will also provide you with valuable tools to shape your life. They will serve as a reminder that you are responsible for the choices you make now that you know about food addiction.

Taking Responsibility

Another reason why many food addicts put off starting their food plan until Monday is responsibility. Food addicts, and most addicts in general, prefer to avoid responsibility, even though they believe themselves to be overly reliable. To an addict, responsibility means accountability. The addict who takes responsibility for his or her actions must then admit to having an addiction. This means abstaining from the addictive substances.

To the food addict, taking responsibility means giving up beloved foods. An addict who refuses to do this is provided with an ever-ready excuse to continue eating. The thinking goes something like this: if I admit I am responsible for my own recovery, then I must begin doing something about it. Quite simply, taking responsibility means leaving the safety and comfort of the addictive world the person has come to know intimately.

Taking action to deal with an addiction also involves some risk, something with which most addicts are very unfamiliar. To an addict, risk-taking is associated with fear. Trying new things means failing in the addict's mind. For most people, risk-taking is difficult, yet manageable. For an addict with a diseased mind, however, the task is completely overwhelming.

One of the major characteristics of addiction, for example, is ritualistic thinking or planning. These contribute greatly to the addict's fear of taking risks. We are not referring to the type of religious rituals usually associated with satanic or harmful activities. We are referring to the type of rituals that make up the addictive person's day. For a food addict, they may involve food, but they may not.

In our research, we have met many addicts who, in a desperate attempt to control their environment, have stringent rules. These include such things as the order in which their clothes should be put on and the types of food they must eat. They are driven by an overwhelming fear of something horrible happening and the pain of an uncontrollable environment. As a reaction, the addict begins to develop rituals in an attempt to ensure future happiness. The absurd part of this is that the more the addict tries to control his or her environment, the less possible this becomes.

In my life, I developed the ritual of putting items in pairs. Whenever I put silverware in the dishwasher, I always made sure there was an even number of items in the holder. It did not matter if I was running late for something important or if something horrible was happening. I always made the time to carefully place the items by twos in the dishwasher.

> I believed that if there were not at least two of each utensil, I was doomed to a life of loneliness and unhappiness. As time went on and I did not see any concrete results, I continued the ritual out of fear. I reasoned that if I stopped this practice, my life would become even more miserable than it already was.
>
> What I did not know was that I had absolutely no control over what would happen to me. It did not matter what way I placed the utensils in the dishwasher. I had created this ritual to have the appearance of control over my world. My fear kept me bound to my ceremonies, making me a slave to their completion no matter what the ramifications.

Overcoming Fear

Other than the physical withdrawal from addictive foods, fear is probably the hardest thing for food addicts to overcome. Addicts are generally fear-based people. For this reason, the topic deserves some additional attention. As you approach chapter 11, you may feel more and more apprehensive about actually beginning a food plan and letting go of your addictive substances.

The most important thing to remember about fear is that 94 percent of the time the thing you are most afraid of never actually happens. How many times have you gotten yourself so worked up over something that did not come true? If it actually did happen by some long shot, was it as bad as you imagined it would be?

How many of your fears are irrational—things that are nearly impossible? Are some of them based on factual occurrences that are blown completely out of proportion? That is another thing about addicts—they have a wonderful sense of the dramatic. This enables them to contrive all sorts of fearful situations in their minds.

Make a list of the things you fear. Do not worry if they seem irrational or silly, just write them down. It does not matter how long your list is or what anyone else thinks. Keep on writing until you feel as if you have gotten them all. When you are done, wait a day or two; then go back and read the list. Be as objective as possible. Pretend that your best friend is telling you these fears. How would you respond? Keep in mind that you probably would not judge your friend as harshly as you would yourself. In other words, do not criticize yourself for having the fear; simply decide how likely it is to happen.

For instance, if you are afraid of earthquakes, consider how many earthquakes you have actually experienced that have injured you or someone you love. Do you even live in a part of the country where they are likely to happen? If you fear losing the love of someone you care about, think about how long this person has been in your life and has loved you. Is this really a rational fear?

When I made my four-page list, I included a fear that I would see someone standing on the balcony of my tenth-floor apartment. After thinking about the probability of this actually happening, I decided it was an irrational fear. Sure, there have been instances where people have done such things, but it was not the sort of thing that happened every day.

After examining your list, pick out the fear that you actually believe may happen. Getting into a car accident, for example, in most parts of the country is a valid fear. Put the fears you have decided are irrational to the side for now. We will discuss those later. Your new list is probably a lot shorter that the previous one. Now, decide how many of your fears on this list involve food, eating, or your body size.

Did you have a lot of fears about losing weight or giving up your favorite foods? Were you afraid of being hungry or starving yourself? Is it scary for you to think about failing at this because it is the last chance you have? Do you fear that your food addiction may be too much for you to handle? Are you afraid of what other people will think if they find out you are addicted to food?

These, and many others, are common fears among food addicts. After years of yo-yo dieting, fears of failing once again are quite strong, as well as fears about being able to manage the addiction. The important thing to remember about fear is that it is a creation of your own mind. Most times, it is based on false assumptions.

Think of fear like this:

> **F**alse
> **E**vidence
> **A**ppearing
> **R**eal

When you are fearing that something will happen, in your mind the possibility is likely. Many times it even seems real. But the reality is that it is a creation of your mind. It is merely a thought you have chosen to give an incredible amount of power to by constantly dwelling on it.

The more you emphasize your fear thoughts, the stronger they become to you. Remember when we told you about affirmations? Fear thoughts work in the same way. The greater the amount of time you spend thinking about something, the more power you give it in your life. In some cases, that which we fear is brought about over the years through the constant attention we provide to it.

Now, take your list and use the same method we gave you to counteract negative affirmations. With each fear thought, for example, think of its equivalent positive message. If you are terrified of not having enough money, tell yourself that you are financially secure and prosperous. Remind yourself that you have everything you need and want.

That which we dwell on increases. It is that simple. Think about something a lot and the power to make it happen increases. Why not think wonderful, productive thoughts to help make your life exactly the way you want it to be?

You've Got to Have Faith

Another effective weapon you have in your battle against fear is faith—faith in the power and order of the universe. We do not necessarily mean the traditional religious faith in God. But if that is what helps you, then use it. We are referring to faith and belief in a "grand plan" for all of us. Belief in a power greater than yourself can help you recover from your food addiction.

For many food addicts, this faith is what saves them when life seems too difficult to face without eating their favorite foods. A concrete belief in the general goodness of the universe is the sort of faith we are discussing. Faith during difficult times will help you maintain your recovery from food addiction.

Self-help, Twelve Step recovery programs, including Overeaters Anonymous, use the concept of a "higher power" in their programs. In these programs, the higher power can be the group itself or traditional religious figures such as God and Jesus. It can also be an undefined spiritual force, an angel, the power of the universe, or even a rock. It is extremely helpful to develop faith in a greater power that will carry you through your most difficult times. Abstaining from your addictive substances will stop the physical cravings for food. To deal with the emotional aspects of the disease, however, a strong faith in a helping force is very helpful.

> When I was first introduced to this concept, I was highly suspicious. I related the idea to the religious financial scandals that were taking place at the time. I was not a particularly religious person and rarely attended church. My only contact with a power greater than myself had come out of desperation. Alone and filled with shame after yet another binge, I turned to God and pleaded for help in losing weight. Since I did not wake up thin the next morning, I was convinced that God did not care about me.
>
> When I began to recover, I saw how unrealistic and selfish my prayers were. I was only concerned with having God remove my weight problem. I never realized the underlying physical and emotional aspects involved. Had God removed all of my excess weight immediately, I would have regained it because I was unaware of my addiction.
>
> Though it did not happen in the time I planned, my weight was removed. And I am thoroughly convinced it happened in a way that is a million times better than I ever imagined. If it had happened my way, I never would have heard about food addiction. And you definitely would not be reading this book right now.
>
> The point is that sometimes I struggle with actually believing in a higher power. When I look back at my past, however, I have a hard time denying its existence. This does not mean that I have become a religious person. I have not. It means that I have developed faith in the universe and my higher power to take care of me when I need it.
>
> That is not to say that my life is perfect. It means that I have what I need when I need it. It is not always the way I want it, but exactly the way it is supposed to happen. With my recovery, I know that I will always be provided with exactly what I need to remain abstinent from my addictive substances.

How do you go about developing this faith? The first and easiest thing for you to do is to stop doubting. Instead of figuring out all of the reasons why you cannot possibly have faith, think about the ways it will help you. Wouldn't it be nice to turn over control of the outcomes of your biggest problems to someone or something else? Imagine the extra energy you would have if you decided to stop obsessing about things.

And even more important, think about how helpful faith could be with your food addiction. Wouldn't it be wonderful to have someone or something to turn to whenever you wanted to eat, no matter what time of day or night? Even better, picture how amazing it would be to have an inner strength and commitment that no one or nothing could destroy. You are suspicious, are you not?

> I had a lot of doubts myself, so I can understand when others have reservations. I always thought that God was too busy or unconcerned to help me with my eating. Why would He care if I ate three french fries? How could I possibly think He would be able to give me strength to deal with my food addiction?
>
> Today, I know that God does help me with food addiction, because I have experienced it. There have been a few times during the past seven years when I have considered eating something that wasn't on my food plan. Usually while I was thinking about the food, something happened to distract me. Sometimes it was a phone call from a friend, a message on television, or a reading I saw that helped. But I know that it was God's way of taking care of me.

This brings us to another way of developing faith—practice. When you get up in the morning, try asking your higher power for the strength to be abstinent from your addictive substances. Even if you do not believe it will help, do it anyway. What have you got to lose? It may take awhile, but if you are persistent in your asking, it will happen. Your life will change for the better. How can we be so sure?

When I first became abstinent, this was suggested to me. I doubted its effectiveness. But, every day when I woke up, I asked for God to provide me with the willingness to do what I needed in order to be abstinent. Then, before I went to bed, I thanked Him for His help during the day. From the first day I asked nearly ten years ago, He has not failed me once.

All of this does not mean that you can simply pray while continuing to eat. Remember, those who help themselves are helped. You have to take the actions recommended in this book in order to be successful. Faith is only one part of your recovery program. Be willing to give faith a try while making an honest effort to abstain from your addictive substances. Follow the other suggestions. Then, you cannot help but be successful.

The easiest rule of thumb to remember about faith is that if you do the "footwork," your higher power will take care of the results. Take the necessary actions to be abstinent—weigh and measure, avoid your addictive substances, use this book, and so on. Then the amount of weight you lose and the quality of your life—the results of your efforts—are up to your higher power.

Other People's Needs

As we struggle with our problems in life, it sometimes helps to have a sense of our place in a larger universe. In other words, try to see yourself as one small part of a much larger grand plan. Addicts, being very self-centered, are often incapable of or have great difficulty thinking about other people's needs for very long. That is unless, of course, they suffer from codependency—addiction to other people.

Before you get upset and angry about our previous statement, read it over. We did not say that addicts don't think about others. We said they did not think about other people's *needs* for very long.

Most addicts will probably contest that statement quite angrily, until they examine their own thinking. Sure addicts think about other people. They think about how they can get other people to help them meet their own needs, instead of considering that others have needs too.

I was thoroughly convinced that I thought about other people's needs. I even thought I put their desires in front of my own until I gave it serious thought. Usually when I did something for someone else, it was to meet one of my needs, not theirs. Giving my friends things, buying gifts for guys I liked, and helping people were all designed solely to meet my needs for companionship and acceptance. I never considered that these people may have needs equally as strong for independence or self-sufficiency.

> More important, I never imagined that whenever I prayed for something I wanted that other people may be affected by it. All I could see was my own selfish need to possess my heart's desire and not my place in a grand plan involving other people. If I had gotten my wish and awakened thin overnight, there are millions of people who would never even know about the disease of food addiction. I have been very vocal in writing and speaking about the disease since my recovery. Would that have been worth getting my needs met?
>
> At the time, active in my disease, I may have said yes. Now I know that what I have today, and what I have been able to give to other people, has been worth the wait.

The point is this: even though you have developed faith, things will not always happen exactly as you want them to. They will happen as they are supposed to, in line with the universe's plan.

All of this may seem a little too metaphysical or spiritual for you. All that's necessary, however, is to be willing to have faith in a power greater than yourself, no matter how you define that. If you believe it will work, then ask a rock to help you with your abstinence. While that may be an exaggeration, the message is there—your belief in a higher power will help you deal with your fears and remain in recovery. All you have to do is ask.

Self-Esteem

In addition to fear, food addicts put off starting their food plans until Monday because they lack self-esteem. As you probably realize by now, the majority of addicts suffer from low self-esteem. There are two basic reasons for this, the first one being the lack of control addicts have over their addictive substances. Food addicts, unable to lose the weight or stop eating unhealthy foods, begin to consider themselves weak, incompetent, fat, lazy, gluttonous, and so on. This causes whatever self-esteem they may have had to disappear. Addicts see the addiction as a moral reflection of their character instead of the disease it truly is.

Addicts also suffer from low self-esteem because of the attitudes they inherited from their addictive relatives. These attitudes of addiction are passed on from one generation to another. Don't worry about how you can increase your self-esteem right now. Simply consider that your low self-esteem may be holding you back from beginning your recovery program.

Food addicts who do not feel good about themselves may not be able to take any action that will allow them to increase their self-esteem. This is due to the uncomfortableness of doing unfamiliar things. While it is difficult to develop new behaviors, it should be noted that it is *not* impossible to change harmful attitudes.

Realize that if you do not like yourself, why would you do things to improve your life? If you had an acquaintance whom you really couldn't stand, would you go out of your way to make this person's life better? Of course not. Your relationship with yourself is somewhat similar to that, with one tragic difference. We have heard many food addicts say, "I would not treat my worst enemy the way I treat myself." What about you? Does that sentence accurately reflect your relationship with yourself? If so, then perhaps your low self-esteem is preventing you from dealing with your food addiction. Start doing things that are good for yourself. "Act as if" you already have high self-esteem. Think about how a person who likes themselves would act. Then do those things, even though it may be difficult. If you are consistent in your "acting as if," then you will eventually develop high self-esteem, which will allow you to treat yourself better. If you pretend that you have good self-esteem, you will acquire it. This will make treating yourself well a way of life. (Chapter 17 describes additional tips on raising your self-esteem.)

As you probably realize, the best way for a food addict to develop high self-esteem is to begin a recovery program, including a method of healthy eating. We know it may not be easy, but we also know it is not nearly as hard as you think it is.

You Will Not Physically Crave Food

The food plan prescribed in this book involves absolutely no magic. There are no hidden activities that you must perform or pills you have to take in order to be successful. It is based on the simple premise that we have described to you about addictive foods. If you abstain from the foods you are addicted to, then you will not physically crave food. It really is that simple. But, although it is a simple idea in theory, it may not be easy. Simple and easy are two different concepts. You probably already understand the notion of food addiction, but right now you are still wondering if you will be able to do this program. This is because you have not begun the food plan, but that is all right. You are simply suspicious about the degree of difficulty involved in the program. We would worry if you were instantly ready to jump into something, anything, without finding everything out about it. That is your right.

And remember that the only way you learn things is to experience them. That is what the next chapter is about—taking the first step to living a life free from the chains of food addiction. Why not give the program a try? It will not hurt you or cause any more pain than you have already experienced. It will be easier than the other methods you have tried. You will not have to constantly count calories. You can eat more than a milkshake for breakfast. You will not have to take pills that have the potential to physically harm you. And you certainly will not have to go without eating for days at a time. You will not be required to purchase special packaged or canned food.

You will not have to starve yourself. And you will not be forced to weigh yourself each week at group meetings. Surgery is not required for this either.

With so little to lose—except of course excess weight—and so much to gain, why not read on? Work at developing your own personal food plan to help you recover from food addiction. Do you really want to wait until Monday to reap such wonderful rewards? Haven't you already waited long enough?

11

Developing Your Food Plan

Here it is—the chapter you have been waiting for. This is the one that is going to help you develop your own food plan based on the information presented throughout this book. Hopefully, you have read each chapter in order and done the suggested activities. If so, you should already have a pretty good idea of what your most troublesome binge foods are. If you've skipped ahead, it may be a good idea to at least read and do the exercises in chapter 9. This will help you identify the foods you are addicted to.

No Counting Calories

So, where do you begin? First, let's examine a few preconceived notions you may have that could hinder the development of a healthy food plan. The most common misguided belief is that it is necessary to count calories to lose weight. When developing your food plan, you should not even think about the caloric value of any food included in your menus. We know at first this may be difficult, especially if you have a long dieting history. After you adjust to the concept, however, it will be freeing to stop determining your meals by the number of calories they contain.

When you give yourself permission to ignore the caloric content of your meals, you will enjoy food more. You will no longer need to look at a chart to create a healthy meal. The reason for ignoring calories is quite simple—they are not an effective measurement of food value for a food addict. Food addicts concerned only with the caloric content of meals may decide one day to eat an entire apple pie for their fifteen hundred calories. And following this system, they may still be able to rationalize the fact that they remained "abstinent" with their caloric intake. This would cause more harm than good. Calories can be used as a justification tool for many food addicts, as well as a method of control. As you probably already know, all calories are not created equally. Four hundred calories of protein is substantially different from four hundred calories of cookies. And it may mean the difference between life and death for a food addict.

Many food addicts, especially those with many failed dieting attempts, also use calories as a method of gaining control over their food intake. This often causes them to become obsessed with the caloric value of each and every food they eat, thus feeding the food addict's psychological obsession with food. Obsessing about low-calorie foods is just as dangerous as obsessing about high-calorie foods.

For a food addict, calories are a meaningless measurement of food in a recovery program. Anyone addicted to sugar, flour, or fats should be concerned only with the ingredients in the foods being consumed. Think of it this way: it does not matter if the food you eat is low in calories. What matters most of all is that it is free of your addictive substances. Low-calorie food high in sugar will cause a sugar addict to binge. This will lead to the intake of much more than the carefully planned low-calorie diet meal.

We know at first this may seem quite unorthodox, but it is important to keep in mind that you are not beginning a diet. You are developing a way of life. While you will lose weight on this food plan, the main purpose of this program is to free yourself from the obsession with food. Think about how many diets you have tried in the past. While you were faithfully following them, what was your main focus? Were you constantly thinking about food? Did you feel sorry for yourself because there were so many foods you weren't allowed to eat?

Traditional methods of dieting, as you read in chapter 2, create a deprivation mode both physiologically and psychologically. Physiologically, if you do not eat enough food, your body works against you in your efforts to lose weight. It confuses your dieting attempts with life-threatening starvation, which decreases your ability to lose weight.

Psychologically, the foods you are prohibited from eating on your diet become the target of your constant obsession. As evidence of this, consider how difficult it is to abstain from eating the foods that you love when you are dieting. If you are like most food addicts, you spent most of your time thinking about the foods you couldn't eat. After a meal, you spent the next few hours resenting the small amounts of food you were forced to eat as your stomach growled violently from starvation. Due to this constant physiological and psychological struggle with your food addiction, you probably stayed on the diet for only a short amount of time.

No Starving Allowed

This brings us to another preconceived notion you may have that will hinder your efforts to develop a healthy food plan. This is the idea that you must starve yourself to lose weight. This myth most likely came about during the time when "crash diets" were first introduced. It is not only harmful to your biological system to starve yourself, but it is also counterproductive in your efforts to lose weight. You may actually lose all of the weight you want in a very short amount of time. But, the minute you resume eating normally—even if that is a healthy amount of food—you will regain the weight.

When developing your food plan, you need to be sure to include sufficient amounts of food. This will ensure an adequate supply of nutrients. The most effective way of losing weight is to omit foods that are unhealthy for you and to eat enough of the proper food you need so you don't feel hungry all of the time. Walking around hungry is dangerous for food addicts. It may, despite any good intentions on the addict's part, cause a binge. Think of eating the proper amounts of food as your insurance against bingeing. If you are full after each meal, you will not need to eat your addictive foods to feel satisfied.

It is like anything else in your life: if you are satisfied where you are, you will not need to look elsewhere for something additional. If you have a job you like, you do not spend your time reading the classified section of the paper. If you are happy with your mate, you certainly are not going to be looking for another. And if you love the place you live in, why would you want to move? It is the same with food once you have stopped using your addictive substances. If you are satisfied with your meals, you are less likely to binge on those foods that could kill you.

No Skipping Meals

Another belief you may need to rethink is skipping meals. At first, it may seem a logical way to lose weight quickly. But considering the ramifications, it is certainly not worth the price. By skipping meals, food addicts set themselves up for a binge. Just as fasting causes an addict to constantly obsess about food until eating becomes the only option, omitting meals eventually leads to the consumption of large amounts of food.

When you skip a meal, you quite naturally become hungry, which may cause you to overeat in the near future. It is very easy for food addicts to think of reasons for eating something not on their food plans. This is especially true during the early stages of recovery when experiencing withdrawal.

Skipping meals, or even portions of them, can become the excuse an addict needs to overeat. Think about how many "rewards" you have eaten when you have done well on your diet or lost weight. For a food addict in recovery, these so-called rewards may be the difference between life and death. There will be enough foods to tempt you without adding to your problems. *It is absolutely imperative, therefore, that you eat everything on your food plan.*

Creating a Lifesaving Food Plan

Take this time to finally erase from your mind the concept of rewarding yourself with food. Instead, view following your food plan as the medicine you need to stay healthy. It is similar to when a cancer patient needs radiation therapy or a person with high blood pressure needs prescription drugs. You need to follow your food plan exactly as it is prescribed without eating more or less. Realize that foods free of your addictive substances, weighed and measured properly, are necessary to your physical health. You need to follow your food plan just as people with other biological illnesses need to follow their drug therapy—in both cases, it's a life or death matter. Sure, your illness may not seem as eminent as the others to you. But, as you have read in the previous chapters, the subtleties of the symptoms of food addiction can be quite misleading. Remember the man who died the night before he was due to be admitted to a food-addiction treatment center? His symptoms were more deadly than even he realized.

It is especially important to keep the idea of eating enough food in mind when you first begin following your food plan. It will be necessary to eat a considerable amount of food on your food plan. Because of this, many food addicts are tempted to declare that there is too much food for them to eat. To this we say, remember all of those binges you had? Is it really too much food, or is it just not the type of food you prefer to eat?

Another preconceived notion you may want to reevaluate is that of eating the same foods daily. Variety is an important element when following a food plan. Boredom may result in an addict seeking additional food, rather than what's on the food plan. Eating the same foods daily may be acceptable if they are enjoyed. Forcing yourself to eat foods you hate daily, however, will only make you feel deprived, angry, and rebellious. This will cause you to reach for those foods you believe will make your life more exciting.

You are not going to find chocolate on your food plan, but it is possible to enjoy a wide variety of good-tasting foods while remaining abstinent from your addictive substances. Also, keep in mind that when your food seems boring, the problem is more likely with your life. In most cases, it is your dissatisfaction with areas of your life that is causing you to consider seeking food as a way of adding excitement to your existence. Instead, realize that variety is the spice of life and the key to success with your food plan. Be creative! Make a whole new dish by combining certain foods on your plan. The end of this chapter contains recipes to help you get started.

Finally, one of the more important preconceived notions you will need to deal with is that of weighing yourself daily. Traditionally, it was believed that weighing yourself every day, weekly at the very least, was helpful. Some programs even included daily or weekly weigh-ins. For a food addict, weighing on a daily basis only feeds the obsession.

For food addicts suffering from high body-image distortions, the numbers on the scale measure success or failure. Considering that weight fluctuates at least five pounds at any given time, this is not even an accurate representation. It is recommended that you weigh yourself only once a month on a set date and time.

It may be tempting, especially in the beginning, to jump on the scale each morning or once a week. In the long run, however, it will do you more harm than good. In the same way that counting calories may become an obsession for food addicts, weight can be equally distracting. Your most important goal when following a food plan should be recovery from food addiction, not concern with your weight. Be true to your recovery program and consistent in following your food plan. Then the other areas, including weight loss, will take care of themselves.

For me, this represented a complete change from the way I once dieted. Prior to getting into recovery, I meticulously planned my weight loss for the following six months. I religiously got on the scale each morning to ensure my progress was consistent with the results I wanted. And when it was not, as was inevitable since my goals were so unrealistic, I would get discouraged.

After that, I would have something special to cheer myself up. It usually started out so innocent. Maybe a cookie or two, I would tell myself. Before I knew it, I had eaten everything in sight. Now, with the food plan I follow today, I no longer have this excuse to eat.

Keeping on a Schedule

This section contains tips that will help you stick to your food plan. First, one of the most important aspects of this food plan is that you eat at about the same time each day. If you have breakfast at 8 A.M. then you should eat lunch between 12 and 1 P.M. Eat dinner around 5:30 P.M. and snack at about 9:30 P.M. to ensure a proper distribution of your food. Minimum time between meals is four hours and maximum is five.

The reasons for spacing your meals are similar to those discussed in the explanation on eating enough food. Not eating meals at regular times can be a setup for failure in the same way that not eating enough food is. By eating meals too far apart, you are putting your body through the feelings of hunger. This may cause you to make unhealthy or destructive food choices. Deciding what to eat when you are in a famished state is dangerous for most food addicts. It is difficult to think clearly when you're hungry.

Eating your meals too close together can also be harmful. When meals are not eaten at least four hours apart, you are not allowing your body to adjust to a set meal pattern throughout the day. If your food plan is executed properly, you will almost never feel hungry, unless you are emotionally upset. The equal distribution of food needed throughout the day will be disrupted unless your meals are at least four hours apart. The food plan is designed to provide you with this. And you will be left with nothing to eat at the end of the day. If you eat all of your food early in the day, you will want more food.

While you may have heard about diets that suggest eating every two to three hours, this is not effective for someone addicted to food unless specific health problems are a consideration. For food addicts already obsessed with food, this is a dangerous idea. Not only is eating eight or ten times throughout the day a means of keeping food prominent in the addict's mind, it is also psychologically damaging to have too much contact with your addictive substance. In other words, the more contact with food, the more danger there is of overeating.

In conjunction with this idea is the notion that all of the food designed for a specific meal must be eaten during that sitting. In other words, it is not acceptable for you to store up all of your protein and eat it at dinner. Physically, you will drastically increase your chances of feeling hungry. Psychologically, you will feed your obsession with food and eating.

Your food plan is designed to help you take your focus off food by discontinuing your use of addictive substances. You will not experience food cravings if you have developed and follow an effective food plan. Why would you want to use another method that would make you obsess about food? Hoarding food for one huge meal will cause you to be preoccupied throughout the day. And you will create an unbalanced food plan.

Say, for example, that you decided to save all of your protein for dinner and not eat any at lunch. Since you have taken food away from your midday meal, you will feel hungry, maybe even angry. Thoughts of your big meal at dinnertime may make you feel better. But, for the entire day, you will think about how wonderful your evening meal is going to be. You will feel excited and happy that you are going to eat so much food. While you are fantasizing about your meal, you are too distracted to concentrate on your daily routine. Instead, all that matters is eating your precious meal. You even decide to eat dinner just a few minutes earlier. You may even think of an excuse to justify why it is necessary.

That night, you are lucky. Even though you ate your meal a little earlier, you were still able to remain abstinent. But, as the days go on, it gets harder and harder. Because you are finding yourself too hungry at lunchtime without your protein, you decide to add a small amount of it to your lunch. This is in addition to your extra serving at dinner. And, since you have done that, you decide that maybe you can have just one extra fruit. You spend hours each day thinking about how you can adjust your food plan to get more food. Eventually, your extra fruit turns into just one cookie which results in a binge. Bingeing brings you right back to where you started, only worse.

Did you see how sneaky the thought process of a food addict is? Switching one serving of protein from lunch to dinner resulted in a binge. The process was expedited for the sake of brevity. But this is the actual cycle that food addicts encounter when they begin taking control of their food plan. Once you have decided on the guidelines of your food plan, it will be most beneficial for you to follow them. Do not alter the formula you have developed.

> While there have been many times when I have been tempted to alter my food plan, I have repeatedly chosen not to. I have seen too many people decide to add a new food or change the amount of something, and then end up bingeing. Through listening to other people, I have learned that taking personal control of my food plan is the first step toward relapse. I equate this to all of the times I had "just one" extra bite of food on whatever diet I happened to be following at the moment. It never ended with that bite, and I believe that changing my food plan would end with the same unfortunate results.
>
> This does not mean that I have to eat exactly the same thing every day. I can change the foods I eat as long as I don't alter the basic plan and the amounts outlined. Over the years, I have determined that the times I most want to change my food plan are when I need to examine what is going on in my life. Wanting to change my food plan is never about needing more food. It is, instead, about a desire for other things that I imagine food may give me, such as security or freedom. Luckily, today I know that this doesn't work.

Weighing and Measuring Food

To follow your food plan properly, you need to weigh or measure your food. We have already discussed some of the benefits of weighing and measuring. Due to the importance of the idea, it bears repeating. Because you are a food addict, your concept of normal portion sizes and your fears about not getting enough food will cause you to misrepresent the amount of food you are allowed. You will either allow yourself too much or not enough food. Weighing and measuring your food is the only way to ensure that you get all of the food you are allowed. You would not want to be cheated out of anything, would you?

When you do weigh and measure, do not skimp. Fill your cup up with vegetables. Make sure your tablespoons are heaping. Think of it this way: if it fits in your cup, it is yours. This also holds true for measuring spoons, though scales are not so ambivalent. Also, be wary of product measurements listed on canned, jarred, or frozen items. You are usually allotted more food. For example, a fifteen-ounce can of green beans will usually fit into your eight-ounce cup.

Think of your measuring tools as your prescription for healthy eating. If you were taking cough medicine, you would measure it out, wouldn't you? Your meals are no different. You need them to survive, as any sick person needs medicine.

> At first, weighing and measuring my food in public was humiliating to me. I felt as if everyone in the restaurant was watching as I put my vegetables into my blue plastic cup. It seemed as if a million eyes followed my movements as I placed my meat on my small white scale. Feeling absolutely humiliated, I refused to make eye contact with anyone for the first several seconds. But, once I looked up, I was amazed to see that not one person in the restaurant was concerned with me or my actions. They only cared about what they were doing.
>
> While I can't say that every time I pull out my cup and scale I am comfortable, I do know that the alternative is not worth the small amount of awkwardness I may feel. If I did choose to give into those feelings and not weigh and measure my food, I would be taking the first step toward my old way of life, and nothing is worth that.

It is also a good idea to develop healthy eating practices. Don't eat as you are running around doing ten other things. Take time to remain seated during your meals and enjoy them. Eat gently and slowly. Throughout the years, many food addicts have developed a love-hate relationship with food. By the time they reach the recovery point, they usually have contempt for food. It is important to realize that it is perfectly okay to take pleasure in your meals.

Don't sit in front of the television. Instead, make time for yourself to enjoy your meals. Put on your favorite music—something soft and gentle. Sit at a table, eating as if you were in a restaurant. It is no longer necessary for you to hide your food. If what you are eating is on your food plan, you need not be ashamed. Your food is perfectly "legal." You are simply taking the medicine you need to live a healthy life, just as a person with high blood pressure would.

Finally, another good idea concerning the development of your food plan is to monitor your thoughts about foods that may become triggers. If you are constantly thinking of a certain food on your plan, it may be a good idea to consider omitting it from your menu. While, at first, this may seem unfair or difficult, consider the consequences. If it really is a problem food for you, then continuing to eat it may eventually result in a binge. Is a few minutes of good taste worth that?

Recovery Is Your Responsibility

The degree of your success in recovery is directly related to the effort and honesty you put into it. No one can do it for you. It is all up to you. If a food on your plan becomes a trigger, you are the only one who can decide to stop eating it. Your recovery is your business and your responsibility.

How does all of this sound so far? It may seem strange or impossible to do or understand, but it is not. It may be difficult to hear about all the work you will need to do, especially when you have never felt any of the benefits. The restrictions seem absurd or unnecessary. Right now, you may not think the efforts are worth the rewards, but how will you really know unless you try?

Perhaps the best gift you can give yourself regarding this food plan is an open mind. As we have discussed before, keeping an open mind allows you to, at least, make an attempt at following a food plan. Even if you are convinced that all of this is garbage, your open-mindedness may cause you to be curious enough to try this program. It is this characteristic that may save your life.

> I am completely convinced that this way of eating is the only reason I am here today. Though I did not have any eminent physical problems when I weighed 328 pounds, it was simply a matter of time before my health deteriorated. My feet were constantly swollen and in pain. My heart raced whenever I walked a few steps. This made me a perfect candidate for any one of a number of health problems, including high blood pressure, heart disease, and diabetes, most of which would have been fatal at my size. By being open-minded enough to try following a food plan, I ended up losing nearly half of my body weight. This dramatically improved my health, extended my life, and allowed me to do things physically that I had only previously dreamt about.

How about you? Think again about the reasons why you picked up this book. Your relationship with food was likely out of control. You probably tried to lose weight a number of times and continually failed. You may be in an enormous amount of both physical and emotional pain. Is this the way you want your life to continue? Isn't it at least worth a try? What if this turned out to be the solution to all of your suffering and you didn't even attempt it? Is that how you want to live the remainder of your life—always wondering what would have happened if you had tried this plan?

As always, the choice is yours, but now the time has come to decide: health or sickness? Those are your two options. When you look at it this way, is there really much of a decision to be made?

The Food Plan

Now, let us begin discussing your food plan. First, we will present a suggested food plan that has proved to be effective for many food addicts. Then we will discuss how you can tailor the plan for your specific needs, including information about how to find alternatives to some of your trigger foods. The food plan we present is a healthy way of eating for anyone, even those unaffected by food addiction. Before beginning, it is, of course, recommended that you consult with your doctor.

Breakfast

The following is an outline of a suggested breakfast plan.

> 1 cup of skim milk
> 1 serving of sugar/flour-free cereal (read serving size on box to determine exact amount)
> 1 serving of breakfast protein (see list for specific items and amounts)
> 1 serving of fruit (see list for specific items and amounts)

Cereals

Any cereal that does not list sugar or flour in the first four ingredients is acceptable. See chapter 9 for a complete list of additional names for sugar. Here are some of the most common cereals without sugar and wheat:

Uncle Sam's	Oat Bran
Kashi	Millet
Grainfield's Corn Flakes	Cream of Rice
Rye Berries	Grainfield's Brown Rice
Puffed Corn	Oatmeal (plain)
Grainfield's Crispy Rice	Puffed Rice
Barley	

The following cereals contain wheat. If wheat is a problem for you, you should avoid them.

Grapenuts	Shredded Wheat
Wheat Bran	Cream of Wheat
Grainfield's Wheat Flakes	Puffed Wheat

Breakfast Proteins

2 ounces (1/4 cup) of the following:

feta cheese	pot cheese (cottage cheese)
low-fat cottage cheese	fish
egg substitute	lean beef

low-fat ricotta cheese   turkey
Canadian bacon   chicken
tempeh

or 1 large egg (limited to three times a week)

or 4 ounces (1/2 cup) of the following:
low or nonfat plain yogurt   tofu

Fruit
Fresh Fruit:
1 whole of the following:
apple   peach
pear   orange

or 1 cup of the following:
blackberries   mango
honeydew   blueberries
Crenshaw melon   cranberries
cantaloupe   pineapple
raspberries   strawberries
mixed fruit

or 2 small of the following:
apricots   bananas
plums   nectarines

or 1/2 of a grapefruit

or canned fruit:
1/2 cup of the following (use only those packed in own
  juices):
apricots   mandarin oranges
peaches   pears
pineapples

or frozen fruit:

1 cup of the following:

blackberries	blueberries
stawberries	honeydew
cantaloupe	peaches
boysenberries	raspberries

You may have an unlimited amount of decaffeinated coffee or tea—provided these are not a problem for you. You are, however, limited in the amount of milk and artificial sweetener you are permitted. If you drink a cup of coffee at breakfast, then you may use some of your milk in it. If you want one at lunch, it must be black, as there is no serving of milk with that meal.

You may also use up to six packets of artificial sweeteners a day, provided they are not a problem for you. If you are triggered to binge by sweet taste, then it will be a good idea for you to omit the sweeteners from your plan. With breakfast, you can also use other condiments such as cinnamon or imitation vanilla flavoring. Be careful with vanilla, as the real one contains alcohol. It is a good idea, however, to limit your servings of both to one teaspoon per day. They may possibly serve to be a problem for you.

Similarly, it is extremely helpful to use other spices if your food is too bland. When making an omelet, for example, add some paprika, onion powder, and a touch of garlic to spice it up, or have some cinnamon in your cottage cheese, or add vanilla to your yogurt for a change. Limit your servings of eggs to three a week, due to the higher cholesterol and fat content. Prepare them with nonstick spray such as Pam or Mazola.

Lunch

Ready to hear about lunch? Remember, schedule your lunch four or five hours after you have eaten breakfast. Your lunch meal should consist of

1 serving of protein (3 ounces females, 4 ounces males)
1 cup of vegetables
1 cup of salad or mixed raw vegetables

1 serving (usually 1/2 a cup) of starch
2 tablespoons of salad dressing
up to 1/2 cup of condiments
1 serving of fruit (choose from the previous listing at
breakfast)

Proteins
3 ounces for women and 4 ounces for men of the following
(weight after cooking):

lean beef (no fat)	chicken
fish	shellfish
lamb	pork
turkey	tempeh
tofu burgers	farmer cheese
low-fat ricotta cheese	feta cheese
low-fat cottage cheese	

or 1 cup of the following:

legumes	kidney beans
black beans	

Proteins may be baked, boiled, broiled, grilled, microwaved, or
stir-fried with nonstick spray. Do not use butter, oil, or fat
when cooking protein. All meats should be lean and not
breaded.

Vegetables
1 cup of the following (either cooked or raw):

asparagus	broccoli
cucumbers	carrots
green beans	eggplant
bell peppers	cabbage
celery	snow peas
tomatoes	cauliflower
radishes	kale
mushrooms	mustard greens
okra	rutabagas

sauerkraut
Swiss chard
scallions
collard greens
dill pickles
bamboo shoots

parsley
water chestnuts
spinach
bok choy
brussell sprouts
onions

Salad Vegetables

1 cup of the following, mixed in any manner as long as they are raw:

arugula
bib lettuce
cabbage
dandelion
mache
radicchio
salad savoy
Swiss chard
watercress

Belgian endive
Boston lettuce
escarole
endive
iceberg lettuce
mustard greens
romaine
spinach

Additionally, any item listed under vegetables may be used in its raw form as part of your salad.

Starches

1/2-cup serving of the following (cooked):

barley
acorn squash
buckwheat
millet
wheat berries
chickpeas
   (garbanzo beans)
black-eyed peas
lentils
split peas
butternut squash

corn
black beans
brown rice*
Kashi
rye berries
black soybeans
kidney beans
lima beans
white beans
peas
parsnips

Others

  4 ounces of potato*
  1/2 ear of corn on the cob
*Potatoes and rice are limited to three servings per week and can be used in either lunch or dinner.

Salad Dressing

Two tablespoons of any salad dressing that does not contain sugar in the first four items listed in the ingredients. It is recommended that you use one that is lower in fat.

Condiments

Sauces:

Up to 1/2 cup of the following, as long as sugar is not listed in the first four ingredients. (You may use together in varying proportions as long as you use only 1/2 cup in total):

barbecue sauce	picante sauce
salsa	spaghetti sauce
tomato sauce	V-8 juice
vinegar	steak sauce
soy sauce	horseradish
mustard	tabasco
tamari	

Other Daily Guidelines:

  No more than six packets of sugar substitute per day
  Up to six lemon wedges per day
  Up to two tablespoons of lemon juice per day
  No more than one teaspoon of imitation vanilla per day
  Up to one cup of clear broth per day with either lunch or
    dinner, if you choose to have it

Spices:

Spices, with the exception of those previously mentioned (lemon juice, vanilla, lemon wedges, and sugar substitute), may be used in unmeasured quantities while cooking. This is provided they do not trigger a binge. While salt is permissible, it is wise to be careful. Limit your use as it can enhance the sweet taste of the substance.

Dinner

Lunch and dinner differ only in that at dinner you do not eat a fruit and you are allowed one serving of fat. This does not mean that you should eat the same things for both meals. It is in your best interest to mix and match items so that you have a nice variety of foods to satisfy your taste buds. Be creative. Mix items together. The following is a list of your dinner foods. Choose from the same listings provided in the lunch section when putting together your dinner menu. Males should double their serving of starch at dinner.

    1 serving of protein (3 ounces females, 4 ounces males)
    1 cup of vegetables
    1 cup of salad or mixed raw vegetables
    1 serving of starch (2 for males)
    2 tablespoons of salad dressing
    up to 1/2 cup of condiments
    1 serving of fat

Fats

1 teaspoon of the following:

vegetable oil	margarine
butter	mayonnaise
olive oil	sesame oil
walnut oil	hazelnut oil

or 1 tablespoon of the following:
    whipped butter
    whipped margarine

Snack

Now that you have made it through three meals, you will be glad to know that you can also eat a snack. It should be eaten before bed. In the event of a late dinner, on rare occasions you may eat your snack in the afternoon. It is not advisable, however, to eat your snack in the morning or midday, as this meal is designed to prevent middle-of-the-night snacking. It should consist of the following:

1 serving of dairy
1 serving of cereal
1 serving of fruit

All of the items should be taken from the previous lists. The only change is the addition of 1 cup of nonfat plain yogurt as your dairy. This is only to be used in your evening snack, and not at breakfast.

Not Enough Food?

So, how are you feeling after reading all of this? It might seem overwhelming at first, but keep in mind that following a healthy food plan is the only way you can recover from food addiction. You simply cannot continue to eat as you have been and experience the benefits of recovery.

Initially, the food plan didn't seem like enough for me. How was three ounces of anything going to be enough to fill me, the one who was used to eating entire half-gallons of ice cream at a time? What good was one cup of vegetables going to do me and who ever heard of eating only four ounces of a potato? I was positive this plan was not meant for me. I was even more certain that it was designed for a slim person, not one who weighed more than three hundred pounds like I did.

When I sat down to my first meal, which happened to be lunch, I was completely shocked at how full I was after I had eaten it. I could not believe how much food I actually got. I also realized that I had no idea how much three ounces or one cup really was. And even better than that, I was amazed at how many delicious-tasting dishes I could eat. This was something I never would have believed if I had not experienced it for myself.

If I had not kept an open mind about trying this food plan, I never would have experienced the incredible benefit. Sure, it may seem like a lot of work at first. But, as with anything practiced over time, it gets much easier. Nearly ten years after my first abstinent meal, I hardly ever think twice about weighing, measuring, and preparing my food. To me, it is just part of the process I go through before I eat a meal. Just as some people cut up all of their meat before they sit down to eat, I weigh and measure my food. What's the big deal?

If you had to take medicine, you would measure that, right? How many tablespoons of cough medicine have you taken over the years? We bet you thought nothing of pulling out a spoon and measuring the proper amount. Try to think of food in the same way. Food is the medicine you need to exist, nothing more, nothing less. Therefore, you must eat a prescribed amount of food each day to remain physically healthy. Your food plan is your prescription, and the food you eat is your medicine.

Food addicts have an advantage over those who take cough medicine. At least they can enjoy what they need to ingest to get better. And speaking of cough medicine, we want to remind you of something very important: if you are truly addicted to sugar, you must be careful when you take any kind of medicine. Read the labels or ask your doctor to prescribe something free of your addictive substances. Many medicines, including cough syrup, vitamins, and aspirins, contain sugar, flour, or caffeine, which may trigger you to binge.

Personalize with Care

With all of this said, we would like to talk about ways in which you can personalize the food plan for your specific needs. Before we do that, know that if you decide to alter this plan, you do so at your own risk. The food plan outlined in this chapter has been proved by many food addicts, myself included, to work for extended periods of time if followed exactly. We have heard about, even met, others who use different food plans. We have also seen or heard of hundreds who have gone back to their old ways once they introduced additional food into their menus.

So, please, be careful, and remember what we said about the

textures of some foods triggering a binge. Food addicts typically turn to these types of foods when bingeing. This means that even though a food may not contain your addictive substances, it could still trigger a binge. This includes such foods as popcorn and rice cakes and any others that are crunchy. Smooth types of food such as cream cheese, peanut butter, frozen yogurt, and applesauce are also dangerous.

This warning does not pertain to those who are altering the plan due to other addictions. If, for example, you find that you are addicted to dairy products, you will need to take necessary steps to take care of yourself. In this case, it is important to make an attempt at the food plan first. If you are allergic to milk, soy milk may be substituted for skim milk.

> At first, I believed I was addicted to dairy items. But, once on the plan, I found it was an addiction to fat that kept me eating these foods. Since all of the dairy on this plan is non- or low-fat, I discovered that my so-called dairy addiction was really a fat problem in disguise.

Make Changes Slowly

If you have decided to experiment with your food plan, do it slowly. For example, if you are convinced that bread and flour are not addictive foods for you, start by having only one serving during the day. See how it reacts in your body. Eat one of the starches listed at lunch, such as kidney beans, but have half a cup of pasta with dinner as your starch. Afterward, notice if there is any difference in the way you are feeling. Did you seem to crave more food after dinner than after lunch? Was your mind clearer during the day, while it seemed "foggy" in the evening?

Monitor yourself for at least a week in this way. If you don't detect any changes, then you can make an informed choice. But remember that if you do introduce flour into your plan, your cravings for it may increase. Since you have discontinued using sugar, your body chemistry has changed. This may cause you to crave twice as much of any brain-altering substance introduced into your system. These are all things you must be aware of when altering your food plan.

Do you notice even small attitude changes about certain food after introducing new items into your plan? If so, it is imperative that you reconsider your decision. Think about how you are acting. After beginning to eat certain foods again, do you have persistent thoughts of being able to eat your binge foods? Are you still living with the hope that just maybe you can eat one cupcake and stop? Haven't you already tried that so many times?

Do you spend a lot of time thinking about the reasons why you should be able to eat this particular food? Have you already eaten more than one serving of the substance at a meal? Are you snacking on it between meals? These are all important questions to consider. Be most honest with yourself. There will be the temptation to rationalize your food choices.

Before making any final decisions about the food on your plan, it may be a good idea to reread the section on rationalization on page 80 in chapter 7. Your denial mechanism is constantly working to keep your eating behavior in a status quo mode. Beginning a food plan is a threat to your denial mechanism; therefore, it will work to keep you from changing your eating patterns. This may mean using such tricks as trying to convince you that just one cookie won't result in a binge. It will try to tell you that you really are not addicted to your favorite foods. At these times, it is very helpful to remember the last time you tried to eat just one of that food. Pull out your eating history as a reminder of your patterns. Are you experiencing anything similar to what happened in the past? Remember, you can prevent binges in the future by learning about the past.

Methods That May (or May Not) Work for You

Now let's discuss a few other ways you can develop an individualized food plan. Some food addicts, though we do not recommend this, follow food plans that do not include weighing and measuring. Instead of using a cup and scale, they will use other means of determining food amounts. A few, for example, will eat a small container of yogurt, a bowl of cereal with milk, and a piece of fruit for breakfast. Lunch would be a plate full of salad with a small can of tuna and one fruit. Two frozen diet dinners would be their evening meal. And they would have a fruit with yogurt and cereal for a snack.

A food plan such as this, however, may result in problems. Many food addicts, unable to consistently judge adequate amounts without the help of measuring devices, will repeatedly increase their portion sizes. If you do decide to follow this type of plan, it is a good idea to use the same plates and bowls every day. This will help you determine consistent serving sizes with your meals. Choose salad bowls for cereal or a dinner plate for other meals, for instance. With this method, instead of using cups and scales as your means of measurement, you will use dishes to keep your portion sizes similar. But, again, it is important to be cautious. This may eventually result in a binge since your meal sizes may vary considerably.

Some warning signs that indicate you are on the verge of a binge include consistently trying to stuff more and more onto your plate as the days pass, eating your meals closer together, spending an increasingly longer amount of time thinking about ways to "beat the system" or eat things not on your food plan, and using larger bowls under the excuse that your usual ones are dirty.

Another way you can create a more individualized food plan is to eat three moderate meals free of your addictive substances each day and a snack at night. This is done without using any means of weighing or measuring your food. It is vital to remember that if you are in the final stages of the disease, this method will not work for you. You will not be able to successfully eat moderate meals on a regular basis without the aid of measuring instruments. In the most serious stages of food addiction, your disease will not allow you to realistically judge appropriate portion sizes on a daily basis.

No matter what your decisions are about your food plan, it is vital that you remember to avoid your addictive substances. Check ingredient lists. Stick to whole foods that you are positive do not contain your problem foods. And, above all else, when you feel drawn to eat your substances, remember the consequences. Once you have reintroduced these foods into your body, you will again begin to crave them. This will most likely result in a binge. It is exactly the same as the alcoholic who is unable to stop drinking once liquor is introduced into his or her body.

If you are truly addicted to certain foods, you will never be able to eat them again without eventually bingeing. While you may not want to hear this, it is important that you realize the truth of the preceding statement. Any doubts you are having at this point may be dealt with by rereading the medical evidence in chapter 2. By now, you may have forgotten the strong documentation presented and a refresher of the material couldn't hurt. Similarly, rereading about other food addicts' experiences in chapter 8 may also assist you in realizing the extent of your addiction.

Withdrawal

When ceasing to eat your addictive substances, you may experience withdrawal symptoms during the first twenty-one days. If you remember other food addicts' withdrawal experiences you read about, you know it is vital that you be prepared for these symptoms. Keeping this in mind will increase your chances for success. You will not have unrealistic expectations about your physical state during the early phase of recovery.

For example, if you feel especially sluggish, have headaches, experience hot or cold flashes, or seem especially irritable, you are most likely going through withdrawal. Your symptoms may differ from those described. And you may not always notice them. But, you will probably experience some sort of withdrawal. The degree of your experience will be determined by the severity of your substance consumption prior to starting your food plan.

Emotionally, it will be necessary to remind yourself that your withdrawal symptoms are not permanent. If you stick with your food plan, you will begin to feel considerably better once your addictive substances are completely out of your system. In other words—hang in there, this too shall pass. When you get discouraged, think about how much better you will feel once you have finished withdrawing. We know that it may seem difficult at times. And because of the nature of addictive people, it may feel more comfortable to reach for food, but doing this will only increase your misery.

One of the best ways to stay on your food plan is to prepare a tasty variety of foods for yourself. It may surprise you to discover the types of foods you can eat on the food plan. For instance, do you realize that you can make chili and still be following your food plan? Or how about a vegetable casserole, or even an Italian bean mixture? And there are many other meals that you can cook. They may even taste better than you ever imagined possible, so before you give up, continue reading.

A Week's Worth of Menus

Following is a week's worth of menus, which are based on the food plan presented in the beginning of this chapter. Recipes for some of the dishes mentioned in the menus will be included at the end of the chapter.

Sunday

BREAKFAST

   1 cup of fresh or frozen blueberries mixed with
   1/2 cup nonfat plain yogurt
   1 1/4 cups Grainfield's Corn Flakes
   1 cup skim milk
   1 cup decaffeinated coffee
   2 packets sugar substitute (for yogurt and cereal or
      coffee)

LUNCH

   tuna (females 3 ounces, males 4 ounces) combined with
   1 cup lettuce, cucumbers, tomatoes, onions,
   1/2 cup chickpeas, and
   2 tablespoons Hidden Valley Ranch with bacon dressing

also: 1 cup sliced tomatoes with
1 tablespoon balsamic vinegar
1 can sugar-free, caffeine-free root beer soda
1 Granny Smith apple

DINNER

lean steak (females 3 ounces, males 4 ounces) cooked with
2 tablespoons barbecue sauce
1 cup Mushroom Mix (see recipes following)
1/2 cup brown rice (females 1/2 cup, males 1 cup) with
1 teaspoon soy sauce
1 cup romaine lettuce, radishes, cucumbers
2 tablespoons Marie's Caesar dressing
1 can sugar-free, caffeine-free cream soda
1 tablespoon whipped butter (for vegetables or rice)

SNACK

1 cup strawberries mixed with
1 cup nonfat plain yogurt
1/4 cup Grapenuts
1 packet sugar substitute

Monday

BREAKFAST

1 cup fresh pineapple
1 scrambled egg cooked in butter-flavored Pam
2/3 cup Shredded Wheat
1 cup skim milk
1 cup decaffeinated herbal tea
1 packet sugar substitute (for tea or cereal)

LUNCH

grilled chicken (females 3 ounces, males 4 ounces)
1 cup artichoke hearts (not marinated)
1/2 cup black beans
1 cup cucumbers, tomatoes, celery, lettuce

2 tablespoons poppy seed dressing
1 can sugar-free, caffeine-free raspberry ginger ale
2 plums

DINNER

hot dogs (females 3 ounces, males 4 ounces)
1 cup Italian green beans
spaghetti squash (females1/2 cup, males 1 cup) with
1/3 cup tomato sauce
1 cup lettuce, onion, green pepper, bean sprouts
2 tablespoons ranch dressing
1 can caffeine-free diet cola
1 tablespoon mustard
1 tablespoon whipped butter or whipped margarine

SNACK

2/3 cup Grainfield's Wheat Flakes
1 cup skim milk
1 nectarine
1 packet sugar substitute (for cereal)

Tuesday

BREAKFAST

1 cup honeydew melon
1/4 cup low-fat ricotta cheese with 1 teaspoon vanilla
3/4 cup Grainfield's Wheat Flakes
1 cup skim milk
1 cup decaffeinated tea
2 packets sugar substitute (for cereal and cheese or tea)

LUNCH

turkey (females 3 ounces, males 4 ounces)
1 cup steamed snow peas and carrots
1/2 cup butternut squash with 1/4 teaspoon cinnamon
1 cup Boston lettuce, dill pickles, mushrooms
2 tablespoons vinaigrette dressing

1 can sugar-free 7-Up
1 bosc pear

Dinner

lean broiled lamb (females 3 ounces, males 4 ounces)
1 cup stewed tomatoes and spinach
Kashi (females 1/2 cup, males 1 cup)
1 cup endive, carrots, bell peppers, snow peas
2 tablespoons sour cream and dill dressing
1 can caffeine-free diet cola
1 teaspoon butter or margarine (for Kashi)

Snack

2 1/2 tablespoons Cream of Rice
1 cup nonfat, plain yogurt mixed with
1/2 cup canned mandarin oranges
2 packets sugar substitute (for cereal and yogurt)

Wednesday

Breakfast

1 cup blackberries and raspberries
2 ounces Canadian bacon
1/3 cup Irish oatmeal with 1 teaspoon vanilla
1 cup skim milk
2 packets sugar substitute (for fruit and cereal or coffee)
1 cup decaffeinated coffee

Lunch

feta cheese (females 3 ounces, males 4 ounces)
1 cup steamed cauliflower
1/2 cup black-eyed peas
1 cup endive, scallions, dandelion, carrots
2 tablespoons Romano cheese dressing
1 can sugar-free root beer
2 apricots

DINNER

1 serving chili (see recipes following)
1 cup iceberg lettuce, cucumbers, peppers, tomatoes
2 tablespoons blue cheese dressing
1 can sugar-free 7-Up
1 teaspoon olive oil for salad

SNACK

1/2 cup canned peaches mixed with
1/4 cup cottage cheese
2 1/2 tablespoons Cream of Wheat with
1/4 teaspoon cinnamon
2 packets sugar substitute (for cottage cheese and cereal)

Thursday

BREAKFAST

1 cup cranberries mixed with
1/2 cup tofu
1 cup Quaker Puffed Rice
1 cup skim milk
2 packets sugar substitute (for fruit and cereal)

LUNCH

canned salmon (females 3 ounces, males 4 ounces)
1 cup cherry tomatoes, onions, snow peas (cold) with
1 tablespoon of vinegar and 2 lemon wedges
1/2 cup black soybeans
1 cup arugula, parsley, red pepper, celery
2 tablespoons Italian garlic dressing
1 can sugar-free, caffeine-free orange soda
1 orange

DINNER

grilled pork (females 3 ounces, males 4 ounces)
    cooked with
2 tablespoons salsa

1 cup steamed asparagus with 1 teaspoon olive oil
acorn squash (females 1/2 cup, males 1 cup) with
1/4 teaspoon cinnamon
1 cup romaine lettuce, tomatoes, broccoli mixed with
2 tablespoons sesame dressing
1 can sugar-free root beer

SNACK

1 cup Grainfield's Brown Rice
1 cup skim milk
1 cup cantaloupe
1 packet sugar substitute (for cereal)

Friday

BREAKFAST

1 cup boysenberries
2 ounces tempeh
1 cup Grainfield's Crispy Rice
1 cup skim milk
2 packets sugar substitute (for tempeh and cereal or tea)
1 cup decaffeinated tea

LUNCH

grilled hamburger (females 3 ounces, males 4 ounces)
1 cup steamed brussell sprouts
1/2 cup barley
1 cup watercress, bamboo shoots, scallions
2 tablespoons poppy seed dressing
1 can sugar-free cream soda
1 peach

DINNER

1 serving Eggplant Casserole (see recipes following)
baked potato (females 4 ounces, males 8 ounces)
1 cup iceberg lettuce, carrots, cauliflower, onions
2 tablespoons sour cream and dill dressing

1 can sugar-free french vanilla cream soda
1 tablespoon whipped butter or whipped margarine
    (for potato)

SNACK

1 cup nonfat, plain yogurt mixed with
1/2 cup canned pineapple
2/3 cup Shredded Wheat with Bran and
1 packet sugar substitute

Saturday

BREAKFAST

1 hard-boiled egg
1 cup blueberries
1/2 cup Uncle Sam's cereal
1 cup skim milk
1 packet sugar substitute (for cereal)
1 cup decaffeinated tea

LUNCH

grilled swordfish (females 3 ounces, males 4 ounces) with
2 lemon wedges
1 cup grilled tomatoes and peppers spiced with oregano
1/2 cup brown rice
1 cup escarole, carrots, cucumbers, scallions
2 tablespoons ranch dressing
1 can sugar-free raspberry ginger ale
2 small bananas

DINNER

roast beef (females 3 ounces, males 4 ounces)
1 cup Italian Stew (see recipes)
Scalloped Potatoes (see recipes) (females 4 ounces,
    males 8 ounces)
1 cup iceberg lettuce, dill pickles, mushrooms, peppers

2 tablespoons blue cheese dressing
1 can caffeine-free diet cola
1 tablespoon whipped butter or whipped margarine
(for potatoes)

SNACK

1 cup nonfat, plain yogurt mixed with
1 cup raspberries, blackberries, cranberries,
1/4 cup Grapenuts and
1 packet sugar substitute

Recipes

The following recipes will help provide variety and good taste while following your food plan. When preparing them, it is a good idea to make extra servings to freeze for those days when you are either too busy or too tired to cook. Then you will have frozen dinners that meet the needs of your food plan. It is also a time-saving and cost-effective means of following your food plan. The recipes are designed to provide at least two servings.

MUSHROOM MIX

2 large peppers
1 teaspoon paprika
10-ounce package fresh mushrooms
1 tablespoon sesame seeds
1 medium onion
1/2 teaspoon dried basil
1 tablespoon garlic powder
1 tablespoon onion powder
olive oil flavored cooking spray

Coat a fourteen-inch skillet generously with cooking spray. Wash and slice peppers, mushrooms, and onion, placing in pan as completed. Add garlic powder, paprika, sesame seeds, basil, and onion powder. Cook over medium heat, stirring frequently and respraying pan when needed for approximately twenty minutes or until tender.

Makes two servings. One cup cooked is equal to one vegetable allotment.

SCALLOPED POTATOES

    5 medium potatoes
    3 tablespoons onion powder
    butter-flavored cooking spray

Scrub potatoes; then cut into thick slices. Coat large cookie sheet generously with butter-flavored cooking spray. Place slices on cookie sheet and sprinkle with half the onion power. Bake at 350 degrees for thirty minutes or until lightly brown. Flip potatoes and sprinkle on remaining onion powder. Bake for an additional thirty minutes or until lightly brown.

Makes two to three servings. A serving (females 4 ounces, males 8 ounces) is equal to one starch allotment.

EGGPLANT CASSEROLE

    1 cup peeled, diced, and cooked eggplant
    1/2 cup tomato sauce
    browned ground turkey
        (females 2 ounces, males 3 ounces)
    1 ounce ricotta cheese
    olive oil cooking spray
    1 teaspoon garlic powder
    1 teaspoon dried oregano

Spray small casserole dish generously with cooking spray. On the bottom of the dish spread 1/4 cup tomato sauce then layer in order: eggplant, turkey, ricotta cheese, and remaining 1/4 cup of tomato sauce. Add spices and bake at 350 degrees for approximately forty minutes or until cheese melts. Makes one serving of both protein and vegetable allotments per meal.

With this dish, you may want to make extra servings and

freeze them for later use. Additionally, other variations of this recipe may be used. For example, try ground beef with tomatoes and pepper instead of turkey and eggplant. You may also use spaghetti squash (females 1/2 cup, males 1 cup) in place of eggplant. If you substitute spaghetti squash, the casserole will count as one serving of protein and starch, NOT as a vegetable.

ITALIAN STEW

1 medium eggplant
2 medium onions
4 medium peppers
2 small yellow squash
2 small green squash
1 28-ounce can tomatoes
10-ounce package fresh mushrooms
2 26-ounce jars tomato sauce
2 tablespoons dried oregano
2 tablespoons garlic powder

Wash, peel, and slice eggplant, squashes, and onions and place in a large pot. Slice peppers and mushrooms and add to mixture along with the canned tomatoes, tomato sauce, and spices. Stir ingredients together. Cook over medium heat for one hour or until vegetables are tender, being careful not to burn the bottom. Divide into one-cup servings and freeze remaining stew.

Makes approximately eight servings. One cup is equal to one serving of vegetables and one serving of condiment per meal.

ABSTINENT CHILI

1 pound lean ground beef
2 small onions
2 28-ounce cans stewed tomatoes
2 15-ounce cans kidney beans
1 large jar tomato sauce
1 teaspoon chili powder per serving

Brown ground beef in skillet and drain fat in colander. Chop onions and brown. In a small covered pot, combine ground beef (females 3 ounces, males 4 ounces), one cup onions, stewed tomatoes, kidney beans (females 1/2 cup, males1 cup), 1/2 cup tomato sauce, and 1 teaspoon chili powder. Simmer ingredients together on low heat for approximately twenty minutes.

Divide the remaining ingredients in the same manner, putting them in individual containers without heating. Freeze the containers for future use. When you are finished, you should have four to six meals. One serving is equal to one portion each of protein, vegetable, starch, and condiment.

TURKEY LOAF

    1 pound fresh ground turkey
    1 small onion
    1 stalk celery
    1 small peeled carrot
    1 small pepper
    1 medium egg
    1/4 cup oat bran
    1 teaspoon garlic
    1 teaspoon pepper
    3 tablespoons soy sauce
    olive oil cooking spray

Chop celery, onion, pepper, and carrot into small pieces. Combine vegetables with egg, oat bran, soy sauce, spices, and turkey to form a loaf on a large cookie sheet or loaf pan sprayed with nonstick cooking spray. Be careful not to leave any hollow spots in the loaf. To prevent this, wet your hands with water and smooth the loaf to eliminate rough areas. Bake at 300 degrees for one hour or until meat is golden brown on both the inside and outside. Divide into individual portions (females 3 ounces, males 4 ounces) and freeze leftovers for future use.

With this dish you can substitute ground beef, tuna, or even ground chicken for the turkey. To give it an Italian flavor, you may also use tomato sauce in place of soy sauce and add 1 tablespoon of dried oregano.

Makes six to eight servings of protein allotment.

Additional Tips

The previous menus were designed as an example of several days' worth of meals. The sample menus illustrate the wide variety of options you have available. They are not intended to be a plan that you follow each week unless you enjoy the foods listed. If you hate brussell sprouts, for example, then you certainly would not want to eat them for lunch on Friday. You will, therefore, need to adjust the menu to suit your own taste buds.

Additionally, do not be too concerned if your budget does not allow for such foods as asparagus or swordfish. You can substitute flounder for the swordfish, or don't even eat fish if you don't like it. It is up to you. There is nothing on this food plan that you must eat if you do not enjoy it.

Similarly, feel free to mix your foods together. The recipes show how you can make some delicious meals with a little imagination. It is very important when combining your foods to weigh or measure each item separately before mixing them together. If you are making chili, for example, the ground beef must be weighed after cooking. Additionally, the cooked kidney beans, tomatoes, and onions must be measured before combining the ingredients. The reason for this is twofold.

First, and most important, separately weighing and measuring each item helps you keep your denial mechanism under control. If you do not weigh and measure your food individually, you may have just the excuse you need to overeat. Without these rigid guidelines, many food addicts find it quite easy to add just a little more of something. You already know this can lead to eating more dangerous foods.

Avoiding Bingeing

Remember, although your addictive substances are not in the foods you are eating, a binge is still possible. There are a couple of reasons for this; the most obvious is that you have used food as a coping mechanism for many years. It is only natural that you would again seek out the substance that you have always used to comfort yourself.

In conjunction with that, during your initial withdrawal period you may find yourself craving your addictive substances. Your body is adjusting to functioning without the aid of these items. When this happens, remember that eating these substances may temporarily relieve your physical cravings. But doing so would only prolong the inevitable withdrawal symptoms. In many cases, returning to your addictive foods makes withdrawal even more severe in the future. Effective ways to deal with these and other similar situations will be discussed in the next chapter.

Weighing or measuring each item individually also ensures that you are eating the proper amounts of food. The success of this food plan depends to some extent on eating specific amounts of food certain times of the day. This is why it is vital to schedule your meals four to five hours apart. Then, you are less likely to binge and more likely to eat the correct amounts of food.

Remember all of those diets you tried that didn't allow you enough food to satisfy a flea? Were you able to stick to them for very long? More important, how did you feel physically? Did you feel rundown and tired most of the time?

You probably felt worse than, if not similar to, when you were bingeing. This is due to lack of proper nutrition in your diet. The food on this food plan is specifically designed to meet your daily nutritional needs. Following the initial withdrawal period of approximately twenty-one days, the plan will make you feel energetic and healthy. This is, of course, provided you do not suffer from additional health problems. Eating too much or too little will disrupt the nutritional balance the plan is designed to provide. This is why it is necessary to weigh and measure items individually.

Try It Now

These recipes and menus are merely suggestions for the wide variety of abstinent meals you can prepare. If, for example, you love green beans, then use them in the Italian Stew instead of the squash. If it is black beans you adore, substitute them for the kidney beans in the Abstinent Chili. Be creative! When doing this, however, be careful to use the proper amounts of each allotment. Do not use one cup of kidney beans to replace the cup of tomatoes and onions in the chili. Kidney beans are a starch while tomatoes and onions are a vegetable allotment. Keep your food plan near you whenever cooking.

> When I first began preparing my food, I kept a copy of my food plan very close so that I could refer to it constantly. Since I had been used to eating whatever I wanted at any time of the day, it took a few weeks to become familiar with the amounts and items listed. As time went on, weighing and measuring and preparing my food began to feel like second nature. Today, it is as natural as breathing.
>
> One of the most useful things I have found when working this program is to have meals in the freezer that I can simply warm up. Like everyone else in the world, I sometimes come home from work exhausted. It is much safer for me to pull out a premeasured meal—usually the chili—that only needs to be heated up than to have to prepare a meal from scratch. This eliminates the excuse of being too tired to weigh and measure my food. With a little planning and time, I have come to realize exactly what I need to have on hand to remain abstinent.

Now that you have read about the food plan, it is more important than ever to keep an open mind. As with any disease, taking the medicine is often the hardest part. Think of this food plan as your medicine. It is not, as you may at first think, a lifetime sentence to eating tasteless food. If this is how you are feeling, reread the menus and recipes. Does this sound like your typical "diet food"? Even more than that, when is the last time you felt totally full while dieting?

The food plan in this chapter is designed to provide you with tasty foods that will satisfy your hunger. While you may have your doubts, it is vital that you be open-minded. At least give yourself a fair shot at recovering from your addiction.

Think the food on this plan is not enough? Well, then, right now, get up, go to your kitchen, and measure out one cup of salad, three ounces of meat, one cup of vegetables, and 1/2 cup of starch. It does not matter what it is for now. Just simply measure out the food. After you have done this, look at the size of the meal. Is it bigger than you thought?

If you are like most food addicts, you have a strong denial mechanism and an overwhelming fear of not having enough food. These two things will cause you to have doubts that the meals on this plan will satisfy your hunger. The best way to deal with this is to do it anyway. When your doubts arise, eat the meal, then see how you feel.

> After over ten years of following this food plan, there are still times when I look at one of my meals and think that it will never fill me. It is the same amount of food I have consistently eaten since I first became abstinent. This happens when I'm very emotional at the time of the meal. When I am experiencing strong feelings, I automatically think of food. Then I start to worry that the amount of food will not satisfy me, even if it's the exact same meal I ate the day before.

No matter what your thoughts about the plan are, you owe it to yourself to give it a try. You have a right to live a life free of food cravings. You deserve that much and more. There is a saying used by Alcoholics Anonymous members that best describes what will happen if you continue eating the way you have been—"If nothing changes, then nothing changes."

Are you ready to change your relationship with food?

12

Just One Bite Can't Hurt, Can It?

Can't wait until Easter, Christmas, or Passover when you can eat all of the foods you love, right? After following this food plan for a while, you will be able to treat yourself to your old favorite foods, right? Wrong! Read on and find out why just one bite of a sugar-filled substance can be deadly for food addicts.

If you are like most food addicts, you are probably trying to think of the next time you will be able to have your favorite sugar- or flour-filled food. You may even be looking at this as just another diet that you will have to endure for a limited amount of time. Maybe you are even planning your next "good meal" after you lose all of the weight you want.

If such thoughts are going through your mind, then it is especially important that you continue reading this chapter even though you may not want to. What you are about to learn may mean the difference between working a successful program and falling into a devastating relapse.

Consequences of Relapse

Remember the personal testimonies in chapter 8? If you have forgotten them, go back and reread them. Pay special attention to those people who discussed the pain they experienced during their relapses. After doing that, think about your own life. Do you really want to go through that? By reading this chapter and the rest of the book, you can at least increase your chances of avoiding a relapse.

It is important that you understand the consequences of a relapse. In chapter 2, you read about how your body reacts to addictive substances, similar to how an alcoholic's body reacts to alcohol. Taking this into consideration, would you say that an alcoholic should be able to have a drink occasionally?

Just like an alcoholic, you will begin to crave your addictive substances the minute you introduce them into your body. You may, if you are lucky, control it for a limited amount of time, but sooner or later—sooner in most cases—you will once again lose control over your eating. This will bring you right back to where you started. In many cases, you will end up even worse off than before.

Is that really what you want? I don't think so. The fact that you have gotten this far shows how serious you are about your recovery. So, read on and find out ways to protect your most valuable asset—your recovery.

There will be many times during your program, especially in the beginning, when you will doubt your addiction. A little voice inside of you will tell you that you really aren't addicted to sugar or flour. It will try to convince you that you can have just one bite. Or, it will tell you that you do not really need to weigh and measure your food. The best analogy we've heard about the strength of your disease during recovery is this: "While you are working hard at recovery, your disease is doing push-ups just waiting for you to eat." The disease of food addiction, whether activated or not, is progressive. Just because you gave up eating your addictive substances does not mean that your body goes back to being in perfect physical shape. Your body will not magically heal itself. The only reason you do not crave your addictive substances is because you are not eating them. You are not cured.

Taking Preventive Measures

Someone in remission from cancer has to take preventive measures to guard against a recurrence. And this person is more likely than someone who has never had cancer to become afflicted again. It is the same for a food addict. And, as with can-

cer, in addition to following your food plan, you can take preventive measures to guard against relapse. The following is a
discussion of those methods.

First, and most obvious, it is vital that you be willing to go
to any lengths to follow your food plan. That means that no
excuse is good enough to overeat. A bad day, too much stress, a
broken romance, a traffic jam, a stalled car, a financial tragedy,
even a death are not, though they may seem so at the time, reasons to eat your trigger food. Because of the coping skills you
have developed over the years, your first reaction may be to
reach for food. This response is so ingrained in your mind that
it may never be unlearned. This means that, scary as it may
seem, relapse begins in your subconscious.

In other words, a recovering person does not have to think
about relapse. It is simply an ingrained reaction process.
Recovery, on the other hand, is a conscious process, one that
must be practiced. Therefore, you need to be constantly aware
of your attitudes and behaviors surrounding food.

What are some of the things to look for? One of the most
obvious is the emotional craving for food. It is natural for you
to want food during times of stress. What about your general
emotional state? If you find yourself especially angry, depressed, defensive, or lonely for long periods of time, it may be
a signal of approaching trouble. Has it been a while since you
felt happy? Are you having trouble laughing?

Other relapse symptoms include a loss of routine, listless-
ness, constantly oversleeping, periods of confusion, increased
irritation with friends and family, irregular attendance at support group meetings, feelings of powerlessness and helplessness, lying, and increased tension. Many food addicts experience
some of these symptoms without adverse consequences. But
the best way to guard against a relapse is to continually be
aware of your emotional state.

Another action you can take to help guard against relapse
is to avoid people and places that endanger your recovery. For
example, you may want to avoid bakeries, ice-cream shops, and
candy stores. The food in these establishments is not on your

food plan and is extremely dangerous to your body. Therefore, you have no reason to even walk through the door. If your family members or friends want a certain item you do not eat, they can get it themselves. If there are children involved and you feel comfortable with it, it may be a good idea to ask another adult to accompany them.

This brings us to an additional way you can prevent a relapse—avoid cooking items that you do not eat. Contrary to what you may think, you do not need to feed the world. It is not a show of strength to prepare your addictive foods. You are not responsible for everyone else's eating habits. You do not have to provide food that you do not eat. With your children or a spouse, you may want to serve their favorite foods, but you are not required to, and it may be a good idea to think twice about it.

Of course, your family and friends do not need to follow your food plan. If you are the person who prepares the meals, however, it may work out that way. While you may want to cook your addictive foods for your family or friends, in most cases, it is not a good idea. Not preparing these foods may even help others in your life develop healthier eating habits.

Would you purposely choose to put your hand in a pot of boiling water? Of course you wouldn't. So, why then, would you consciously choose to handle food? Whenever you touch something that you do not eat, it is like handling dynamite. It could explode at any moment, and for a food addict that could mean a devastating relapse.

Avoiding extremely stressful situations is another way to prevent relapse. In today's fast-paced society, it is virtually impossible to avoid all stressful situations. However, if you are like most addicts, you may be creating them without even knowing it. For instance, how many times have you agreed to help out or go with someone when you really did not want to?

We all have obligations in our daily lives—that is inevitable— but how many of them truly are necessary? Aren't there things in your life that you could stop doing if you really wanted to? We are certainly not advocating becoming a hermit. We are saying it is very important to choose the activities that you commit your time to carefully. Your first obligation has to be to yourself and your program. If it is not, you will not be in any shape to help others.

Making Changes

After getting into recovery, many food addicts have to change certain aspects of their lives to remain successful in their programs. If, for example, you are working as a food server, you may want to rethink your career choice. We are not saying you can't be a food server. But we do think it is vital that you honestly look at how your job could negatively affect your program. In some cases, it will not. We know of food addicts who are able to serve food without any problems. That is not true for everyone.

We have heard of many food addicts, for instance, who have had to modify their entertaining habits. There are those who used to cook for everyone in the neighborhood, for instance. Continuing this activity will most likely not allow them time and possibly the desire to prepare their own meals.

> I used to bake chocolate chip cookies for everyone in my neighborhood at school. After getting into the program, the stress of smelling the cookies and my newfound knowledge about my addictive substances caused me to reconsider my decision. Since I began following my food plan, I have baked cookies a few times and that was later in recovery. Before that, I did not feel strong enough to smell them and did not want the stress involved.
>
> It is important to remember that everyone is different. You may be able to bake cookies. The important thing is to be completely honest with yourself where food is concerned. The best rule of thumb I have heard is this: "When in doubt, leave it out." This can apply to foods you are unsure about as well as activities about which you are undecided.

Now, we would like to discuss a few more ways you can avoid stress that does not involve food. First, examine your job. Is it something that you like to do or can, at the very least, tolerate? If not, then at some point you may want to consider changing jobs, maybe even careers. It is preferable to wait until you have been working your recovery program for at least six months to avoid rash decisions. Stress from your job can be dangerous. If, for example, you are working ten and twelve hours a day, when do you think you will find the time to prepare your food? While it is possible to remain in recovery with such a demanding schedule, we do not recommend it.

> A few years ago, I was working a job where, in order to beat the traffic, I had to leave my house at 7 A.M. I did not return until at least 6 P.M. After sitting in frustrating traffic jams for more than an hour, I had no desire to prepare dinner when I got home. My commitment to recovery was strong, however. To deal with this, I prepared a week's worth of meals each weekend. When I got home each night, all I had to do was pull a dish out of the refrigerator and heat it up in the microwave.
>
> After more than a year of doing this, however, the stress became overwhelming. I found myself angry and resentful about having to give up my precious time off to prepare the entire week's worth of meals. And coupled with my other commitments, which include attending support group meetings, exercising, and writing, cooking this amount of food left me completely stressed out and overwhelmed. My life was so full that I did not have time for fun. I could not even make plans on the weekend without preparing for weeks in advance in order to have time to cook my meals.
>
> Realizing that I could not continue in this manner and remain successful in my program anymore, I had to make some choices. And I knew they were not going to be easy ones to carry out either. My job seemed like a good career move on my part, and I was making a decent salary, enjoying some of the finer things in life. Yet, I knew that the absolute, most precious thing I had was my recovery. There was nothing more impor-

tant to me than protecting that. I knew everything I had achieved in my life happened because I was coherent enough to go after it.

Choosing my job over my recovery, to me, meant that I would lose everything. If I kept working at it much longer, I knew my recovery would suffer, and I would soon be eating my addictive substances. If that happened, I would be in a drugged state which would cause me to make mistakes at my job that could eventually result in termination. From my past experience, I realized that my success in the job depended on my being functional. And when I eat my addictive substances, I am not able to concentrate on anything except food. Even with flawless reasoning such as this, I was still unsure. The economy at the time was in bad shape, and finding another job would not be easy.

After months of contemplation, I decided that I was willing to take a risk with my financial situation but not with my recovery. I quit my job without even having another one. I had gotten to the point where I couldn't wait any longer. The pain was too overwhelming. At the same time, I went through a period of reevaluating my career choice. I realized that my true passion was and is writing—a choice that I had put aside during my binge-eating days. With all the changes taking place in my life, I decided to follow my dream, though I knew it would not be easy.

A week after leaving my job, I got a part-time position at a local college, which allowed me more time to write. Since then, there have been both easy and difficult times financially. But, as far as my recovery is concerned, I have continued to abstain from my addictive substances. In addition to this, I have taken concrete steps to make a lifelong dream about my career a reality. I have also eliminated tons of stress from my life, which has caused me to continue successfully in my recovery.

The point of this story is to show you that even situations that seem overwhelmingly stressful can be eliminated, though this may seem impossible at the time. We are not advocating quitting your job as a means to a more successful recovery. We are merely providing you with an example of how stress can be extremely dangerous to your program. But, once again, the choice about where and how to eliminate stress from your life is up to you. We can only outline the framework for making those choices. We cannot make them for you, as only you know your needs.

HALT Method

The topic of stress also brings us to another important method for avoiding relapse. It is best summed up by Twelve Step programs in the following:

Try to avoid getting too

Hungry
Angry
Lonely
Tired

when working your recovery program. This is known as the HALT method.

Using the HALT method is an effective way of preventing relapse. When food addicts become too emotional, as we have discussed, their recovery program is at risk. The emotions of hunger, anger, loneliness, and tiredness are those from which addicts are most likely to need consolation. And in the past, most food addicts sought consolation through eating their addictive substances.

A good way of using this method is to HALT whenever you start feeling yourself fall into these emotions. If you have gone more than five hours between meals, you will need to HALT what you are doing and eat. If you find yourself becoming unusually angry about something, HALT and remove yourself from the situation. When you start feeling overwhelmingly lonely, HALT what you are doing and take steps to change your situation. Call a friend or go out and have fun. If you have become too tired, HALT and get some rest. Remember that you are not superhuman. Your body has certain physical needs, and it is important that you listen to them. The HALT method is a good reminder of ways to keep your recovery program in check, thus avoiding relapse.

Sharing with Others

Still another effective way to avoid relapse is to share your recovery program with someone who understands. (Information about support groups and additional recovery methods will be provided in chapter 14.) Sharing your experiences helps prevent your feelings from becoming overwhelming, which may lead to a relapse.

Most food addicts have difficulty communicating their needs, desires, and feelings to others. An important element of any food addict's recovery is learning how to express feelings. When choosing a confidant, it is important to select carefully. While your first reaction may be to turn to old friends or family members, first consider the ramifications of your choices. You will be sharing many parts of your personal life, as well as your food history, with this person.

Choosing to speak with your child about your difficulties with parenting, for example, may not provide either of you with a healthy, supportive environment. At some point when you are calmer, you may choose to discuss your past mistakes with your child. During the initial phase of recovery, however, it is a good idea to find someone you have more in common with to discuss your feelings. This example may be an obvious one, but it is effective in making the point about choosing carefully the person you confide in.

It is also important to note that sharing your feelings with someone who is incapable of understanding them will only cause you pain. Deciding to tell your friend who is still using his or her addictive substance about your feelings of sadness over giving up certain foods will only fall on deaf ears. Your friend has no frame of reference to relate to. Because of this, it is vital that you develop a support group you can turn to when you need to share how you feel. And these may not always be sad or upset feelings either. For many food addicts, extreme happiness and joy are equally hard to manage. You will, therefore, want to choose people who are able to relate to both your ups and downs.

If you are not ready to share your feelings with other people, then try keeping a journal of your emotions. It does not have to be anything fancy. An old notebook will do. Just pick up a pen and write down how you are feeling. If you don't know, then write that. Write anything that comes into your mind. You don't even have to do it every day as long as you write on a fairly regular basis. Keeping a journal will provide you with an outlet for your feelings. Writing is especially helpful if you are having a hard time talking about your feelings. Remember, it is important to get your feelings out before you have problems.

Interrupting Relapse

What should you do if you notice yourself slipping? Your main objective should be to interrupt the relapse and return to recovery. The following are several steps you can take to accomplish just that.

First, list the warning signs you have noticed. What do you think is causing them? Try to figure out what your problem is. You may already have some idea, but once you examine it in detail you may discover surprising new things.

For example, if you have been really depressed and unhappy about the way your relationship is going, it may signify something deeper, a dissatisfaction with your own life. Even if there is nothing deeper, writing down your problem will help you to be clear about what is happening to you. This will, in turn, allow you to begin taking action to solve your difficulty.

After you have discovered your problem, make a list of at least five possible solutions. What can you do to solve what is happening to you? All too often, food addicts, bound in their fears about change, remain tied to one solution. This means they neglect the wide range of options available to them.

> With my job problem, I listed alternative ways of making money, which included taking in a border and typing resumes. Making the list did not commit me to doing any of the activi-

ties. It only helped me to determine my options. And once I saw how many choices I had, it was easier to take such an overwhelming step.

Once you have identified your options, ask yourself three questions about each: (1) What is the best possible result if I choose this remedy? (2) What is the worst possible result if I choose this option? (3) What is the most likely result from this solution? Next to each option, list your answers to the questions.

Review your options and the answers to the previous questions. Then, choose the remedy that will most likely help you interrupt the relapse process and take action. Try not to listen to your fears. Instead, think of what you need for recovery.

> Quitting my job, though one of the scariest choices, was the best way for me to prevent a relapse. This was especially true once I noticed several of the initial warning signs.
>
> For the first time in my recovery, I was waking up depressed. I didn't want to start the day and I hated my life. I was beginning to feel as hopeless as I did before I became abstinent. That's when I knew I had to do something. Nothing was worth the pain of going back into my disease.

Following the action, evaluate the results. How has it worked? Have your relapse symptoms disappeared? Are things better for you? Do you still feel as you did? If your situation has improved, congratulations! You have probably successfully diverted a devastating relapse. If no improvement is made, you may want to go through the previous steps again or develop a new course of action. Either way, you are on your road to recovery as long as you are willing to continue taking the necessary steps.

What to Do If You Relapse

It does not matter what course of action you take to prevent a relapse. The only thing absolutely necessary is that you remain willing to work on your recovery. No one method is perfect for everyone, and you may find other things that work better for you. It does not matter what it is, as long as you are comfortable with it and it does not harm others.

Perhaps the most vital thing to remember when working your recovery program is that you have a disease. If you should relapse, the best thing you can do for yourself is to refrain from blaming yourself. As with cancer, you may experience a relapse in your recovery, but it is not your fault. Sometimes you may be able to complete the exercise mentioned and come out with concrete solutions to your problem. But other times, there may be no reason for your relapse other than the fact that you suffer from a chronic disease.

This is not to say, however, that relapse must be a part of your recovery program. It is possible to enter recovery and stay there indefinitely. We have heard of people who have been in recovery for as many as ten or twenty years.

> I know it is possible to stay in recovery. For the past ten years I have been working my program without a relapse, and it still amazes me. When I started, I didn't think I'd even make it through one meal, never mind a day. It can happen to you, too, but if it doesn't, keep working at it and it will work.

If a relapse does happen to you, it is a good idea to look at it as a learning process. When you come out of it, and even while going through the relapse, realize that you are learning valuable lessons about yourself and your recovery program.

It is also important to remember that no matter what may happen with your food, you do not want to add to your distress by continuing to overeat. Unlike the dieting you've done in the past, this program is not a matter of being "on or off" the diet; it's about living a sane life. If you do begin to eat sugar, for example, remember that you have a choice. You can stop at any moment and continue on in your program. There is no need to wait until the next day. Don't add to the mistake by allowing yourself to continue bingeing.

Perhaps out of this trauma came more knowledge about

yourself or an even greater commitment to your recovery program. Maybe you discovered exactly how addicted to certain foods you are or even that you truly are addicted. Whatever it is, it is important that you are aware of what you have learned and that you do not punish yourself for relapsing. Beating up on yourself will only cause you more pain than you have already experienced. Is that what you want?

Finding a Higher Power

Before closing this chapter, we would like to discuss one additional way to prevent a relapse. We have saved it for last because it is probably the most difficult and controversial method you have read about thus far. For many people this becomes a last resort, thus its place in the chapter. While we briefly mentioned it before, it is important to cover it in greater detail at this point. The method involves developing a belief in a power greater than yourself.

In previous chapters, we discussed the reasons for the importance of this. To briefly review, developing this belief is vital to your program. It provides you with someone or something stronger than yourself to rely on during difficult times. No matter what your choice of a higher power is, you need to develop a working relationship with it. This can be as simple as asking for help when you feel like eating or as extensive as establishing daily contact with your higher power. But either way, developing this relationship is an effective way to prevent relapse.

> Coming from a childhood of little or no spiritual beliefs, I had a difficult time establishing a relationship with a higher power. The most effective way I have found is to simply pretend that there is a higher power looking out for me. So, when things get difficult and I feel the urge to eat, I simply look up and ask for help in dealing with the situation. And for more than ten years that has worked.

Your higher power, however, is not going to take the food out of your mouth, and it will not make you thin overnight.

Instead, your help will come in small ways as you continue to follow your program. This book, for example, is a way your higher power may have chosen to help you with your food problem. Even if you put this book down and do not look at it for another two years, the seeds have been planted. And in time they may blossom into a wonderful new life.

We hope this chapter has provided you with some effective ways of preventing and dealing with relapse. It is important to note, however, that professional help may be needed to deal with certain situations. In the next chapter, you will discover how to say no to well-meaning family members and friends who may inadvertently attempt to sabotage your recovery program.

13

No Means No!

Sure, the food plan sounds great, and maybe you are convinced that you will be able to follow it for a while. But what happens when you see your favorite food-pushing relative? How can you possibly say no to the food without hurting this person's feelings?

This chapter will provide you with ways to say no and remain on your plan. You will be instructed in boundary-setting and effective communication skills designed to protect the program you have worked so hard on. Before you go out there in the real world, finish reading this chapter and learn how to take care of yourself and your program.

The first and absolutely most important thing to remember about saying no is that "no" is a complete sentence. Period. End of discussion. While in some cases you may choose to offer an explanation for your refusal, it is not required. The key words in the previous sentence are "you may choose to offer."

Most food addicts go out of their way to make up excuse after excuse about why they have said no. This is because of the codependent nature of the addiction. Addicts naturally tend to try and please other people, to be liked and accepted—a feeling they have never experienced toward themselves. Instead of looking inside themselves for validation and self-esteem, most addicts look to other people and outside experiences, with the mistaken belief that outside sources are responsible for creating good feelings about themselves.

Your first response to an invitation to eat something, therefore, is most likely to be an automatic yes due to years of programming. How many times have you just automatically said yes when someone offered you food? Even if there was a rare instance when you did not want any food, you probably still used the excuse that you would hurt their feelings if you said no.

Think back to last week or last month, the last holiday, or even yesterday. How often have you said yes to something—not necessarily food—when you really wanted to say no? If you are like most food addicts, there are too many instances to remember. How can you change your yes into no without hurting others?

First, realize that, cold as it may sound, your refusal to eat or do something may hurt someone else. And if it does, that is their problem, not yours. While you should not purposely hurt other people, realize that it is impossible to please everyone all of the time while still taking care of yourself. And you should not try. Did you hear that? *You should not try to please everyone.*

Trying to please everyone is the easiest and quickest way to put yourself right back where you started, maybe even to a worse place. But, how can that be? Aren't you *supposed* to be nice to others? The answer is yes, of course, being nice to others is a good idea. Trying to please everyone, however, is not. The fine line between being nice and trying to make everyone happy is one that is unclear to most food addicts.

Setting Boundaries

This is where the concept of boundaries comes into play. Boundaries are exactly as the name implies—limits on the behavior you will and will not accept. Unfortunately, setting boundaries does not mean you have the ability to control another's behavior. It is only a way of defining your limits. For example, you cannot stop an overweight family member from overeating. You can, however, refuse to either contribute to the behavior or be around it. Doing those things means you are setting your boundaries.

When you set boundaries, you are standing up for your

rights, which helps you to respect yourself and other people. Sound a little strange to you? Think about it this way: putting limits on the behavior you will accept from others shows that you are concerned enough to take care of yourself. It is like caring for your most precious possession. Take your car, for example. Whenever you wash or polish it, you are helping to preserve its beauty. It is the same with you—setting boundaries helps preserve your magnificence.

So, how do you do it? The easiest and most effective way to set boundaries is by using "I" messages. Most people are all too familiar with "you" messages—you hurt my feelings; you made me angry; it is your fault I am lonely.

"I" statements are exactly as they imply: messages that describe what you saw, felt, or heard, which label your feelings. By using the "I" model, you are taking responsibility for your feelings. Saying, "I feel hurt when you criticize me" is quite different than, "You hurt me with your criticism." Can you recognize the difference? The one using the "I" message paves the way for nonthreatening, open communication, while the "you" statement may result in aggressive, argumentative reactions.

Think about how you feel when someone directs a "you" message at you. Do you get angry? Defensive? Combative? Does it feel more like an accusation than a way of communicating? More important, when a "you" message has been directed at you, does it make you want to continue discussing your feelings with the person who said it? Of course not. Instead of opening the lines of communication, "you" statements pose the receiver for combat.

Now that you have got the formula for stating your feelings in a nonthreatening way, let's discuss your delivery. The manner in which you express your feelings is as important as the words you use. For example, an "I" message said in an insulting, angry tone is as much of a communication block as any "you" statement.

How do you deliver a calm, nonthreatening "I" message when you feel as if you will explode? The best answer to that question is this: you do not. That is not to say you don't express your feelings. Instead, you simply wait until you are able to state them calmly. For some people, it only takes a short trip to the rest room. For others, it may require days of contemplation before being able to share their feelings. Whatever it takes is whatever it takes. There is no statute of limitations on expressing your feelings.

In addition to using "you" statements, there are other ways that many food addicts unknowingly block communication. Perhaps the most popular method used is advice-giving. Think about the people in your life. Is there one who always seems to know exactly what is best for you? A person with all of the answers? How does it feel when the advice is directed at you? Does it make you want to share your feelings with this person? In most cases, the conversation will result in a one-sided sermon instead of an open discussion about feelings.

Another block to communication is interrupting. Having an open conversation about feelings is nearly impossible if one person constantly blocks the other's attempts to participate in the discussion. Sharing your feelings is as much about talking as it is about listening. So, the next time you are involved in a conversation, notice how many times you interrupt the other person.

Open Communication

Another barrier to open communication most food addicts use is to always agree. While at first glance this may seem like a way of opening the lines of communication, it does exactly the opposite. By constantly agreeing with someone during a conversation, you are preventing the other person from knowing your true feelings. Hiding behind a barrage of yes answers causes distance and ultimately a one-sided conversation. Discussing your true feelings about any subject, on the other hand, opens the lines of communication.

Other communication blocks include mumbling, avoiding eye contact, daydreaming, fidgeting, name-calling, changing the subject, preaching, using lofty words, constantly apologizing, walking away, and screaming.

How many of the blocks did you recognize from your conversations? Remember, the point of learning about these things is simply that—to learn, and not to beat up on yourself. Just because you are in recovery does not mean you are expected to be perfect. Quite the contrary, once you enter recovery your learning is just beginning. Prior to this, when you were active in your disease, you were too preoccupied with food and eating to be aware of your actions. Now, and for the rest of your life, you have the time and, more important, the ability to discover more about yourself.

Begin by recognizing your communication patterns and slowly work on improving them. It is not necessary, nor a good idea, to try and change your entire life in a few weeks. As with your entire recovery program, small, concrete steps are much more powerful than huge, thoughtless ones.

A Twelve Step program slogan best describes the attitude you should approach your program with: "Easy does it, but do it." Therefore, fifteen minutes a day of doing something to strengthen your recovery is much more potent than cramming eight hours of recovery into one day per week. Preparing your food for a few minutes each day is more effective than sticking to your plan only on weekdays.

Assertive versus Aggressive Behavior

Now that you understand what blocks communication, we would like to point out the differences between assertive and aggressive behavior. This will further help you in expressing your feelings. We will start with definitions of the two. "Assertive behavior" is taking action in a respectful and understanding manner to fulfill your needs; it helps promote and maintain positive, constructive relationships. Think of it this way: assertive behavior is stating what you need and want in a non-threatening way. Applying this analogy to your car, assertive behavior is polishing the car, changing the oil, and generally maintaining the integrity of the automobile.

"Aggressive behavior," on the other hand, is expressing feelings in a manner that threatens, strains, or harms a relationship.

Applying it to your car again, aggressive behavior is slamming the door of your car, constantly speeding, and ignoring the car's mechanical needs. Examples of aggressive behavior include manipulation, sarcasm, spitefulness, attacking, and hurtfulness.

Do you see the difference? Aggressive behavior demands answers or actions while assertiveness states needs and wants. Let's take an example of a situation and examine three different reactions to the occurrence. The situation: your spouse comes home drunk and wants you to stay awake late into the night when you have to get up early for work the next morning.

Three Examples

In the first example, you quietly mention that you are not able to stay up due to your work schedule. You do not want to hurt your spouse's feelings by saying that you do not enjoy being together during these times, so you remain silent. When your spouse protests, you eventually give in and grudgingly stay awake for three hours longer than you had planned. This leaves you tired and unable to perform adequately at work the next day. After a grueling day at work, you return home and quietly sneak away to your room where you spend the rest of the evening sleeping.

In the second example, you calmly but firmly tell your spouse that you feel hurt and angry about the situation. You say that you love your spouse but you are not able to stay up late due to your work schedule. When your spouse protests, you restate your feelings and head for the bedroom. The next day, you awaken refreshed and ready to tackle the demands of the day ahead.

In the third and final example, you greet your spouse with the words, "You are drunk." Though your voice is calm, your words are cutting. When your spouse asks you to stay awake, you laugh loudly saying that you have a job to go to tomorrow. You remark that unlike some people, you cannot afford to stay up all night. Your job is too important for that. When your spouse protests, you begin a ten-minute dissertation about how many sacrifices you have made in the relationship. After stomping off to your room, you slam the door and awaken the next morning slightly tired but ready to meet your work demands.

Which reaction do you think is the best way to state your needs and feelings? If you said the second one, you are correct. The first situation is an example of what is known as "nonassertive behavior," which is similar to the "people pleasing" discussed earlier. In this case, you are avoiding taking responsibility for discussing your feelings. You are living with the hope that someone will guess what you want and need instead of taking action.

And, in the final example, aggressive behavior was used. Instead of calmly stating your feelings or needs, you used accusations and insults. You bullied your spouse into trying to see things your way. At the same time, you avoided discussing your feelings. In this case, though you are more vocal about it, you are still not telling your spouse what you need or want in the relationship. This type of action actually damages the trust in the relationship.

In the second example, by using assertive behavior you accomplished several things. First, and most important, you clearly stated your feelings. This will help you to avoid holding on to a resentment that may cause you to turn to food in the future. Remember, when you keep your feelings locked inside, they grow and may eventually become so overwhelming that you seek consolation in the same way you always have—eating.

By applying assertive behavior, you also maintain the integrity of the relationship. In this case, trust and open communication are preserved. This means that you and your spouse will be able to continue talking to each other openly and honestly and will respect each other's feelings. In other words, you come together as two equals.

When improving your communication skills, it is important to remember that things are not going to change overnight. Be patient with yourself and celebrate your small accomplishments. And no, we do not mean by eating. Notice your progress and do something nice for yourself to recognize it. Go to a movie. Take a long, hot bath. Or snuggle up with a good book. Do something just for you.

So, what does all of this have to do with saying no to well-meaning family members or friends who constantly offer you food? By learning to be assertive instead of aggressive when you are offered food, you will be able to say no to them. In most cases, you will not even cause an argument.

Just Say No

Now you have a basic idea of the difference between aggressive, assertive, and nonassertive behavior. Next, we will present some specific examples that will help you to say no to family or friends. The first one involves your grandmother. After explaining the details of your new food plan to her, she offers you some home-baked chocolate chip cookies. Your first response is to get angry. You might even say mean things to her about how she did not hear a word you said, but you know better.

Instead, you calmly tell her, "No, thank you, Grandma. I explained to you that I do not eat sugar or flour anymore. It is not healthy for me." You can stop there if you choose to or you can continue to discuss the situation. If you continue, be gentle and keep your statements in the "I" form. A no answer to cookies that she worked on baking all day may be more than Grandma can handle at that moment. Remember, there are two sides to every conversation. Grandma may be feeling rejected because this is the first time you ever refused her cookies. New behavior methods are difficult for both the initiator and the receiver. That does not mean you should avoid using them; it only means to start out slowly. If, after several times of saying no to Grandma's cookies and explaining your feelings, she persists, it may be time to realize that Grandma is not going to change. In this case, you must make a decision. Can you continue to visit Grandma and face her offer of cookies? Are you in a strong enough place to resist or do you need to limit frequency of your visits? If you do decide to cut down on your visits, know that, after a few months, you might be stronger and more able to handle seeing her on a regular basis. No decision is carved in stone.

When faced with such a situation, just be sure to make the decision based on your needs and not on anything else, such as revenge or people-pleasing. Doing this will not help either one of you. No matter how much of an actor you think you are, Grandma will, most likely, be able to pick up on your resentful attitude.

What do you do with the guilt you feel about not seeing her? The first thing to understand about guilt is that it is your problem. No one else is making you feel guilty. Instead, you are allowing yourself to feel guilty. It may be a pattern set up during your childhood, but you are not a child anymore. You have the right to choose whether or not you buy into the old messages you were sent. While you cannot immediately stop yourself from feeling guilty, you can take steps to lessen the feeling until it eventually disappears.

Writing about your feelings, for example, will help you to release them. It will also allow you to objectively look at exactly what you are feeling and why. Write down all of those horrible thoughts that are going through your mind, the ones telling you how awful you are. Then, reread them a little while later, or even the next day. Is this what you really want to believe about yourself? If possible, ask a friend about them. Does your friend consider them true? You may even want to discuss them with a professional.

It may also be helpful to examine your guilt. What is the reason for it? Think about the messages you give yourself. Are you under the impression that other people's happiness depends on you? Or, are you feeling guilty because you are trying to please someone else by living up to their standards? Even more serious, are you using guilt as the excuse to repeat the behavior? Do you continue visiting Grandma, for instance, so that eventually you can use her insistence that you eat cookies as your rationale for eating them?

Think about that last question very carefully. Isn't that a

convenient excuse for overeating? "My grandmother made me do it!" How could you possibly be expected to resist such a cute, little old lady? After all, you don't know how much more time she has left on this earth, right? You would not want to be the one who pushes her over the edge by refusing to eat her cookies, would you?

Can you see how this thinking works? By blaming Grandma, you have given yourself permission to eat not only the cookies, but anything else she offers you. You have also justified your actions by using Grandma's health and old age as an excuse. This is exactly how your disease works. It will do anything it can to get you to eat. But the ultimate choice is yours. Do you really want to return to the way it used to be?

It is vital to remember that no one can make you eat. And it is no one's fault if you do eat something not on your food plan. There is no person, situation, or occurrence that can make food jump into your mouth. And that includes Grandma.

Your Rights

Also, remember that it is your right not to eat your addictive substances. You have the right to say no to anything that is not healthy or good for you. You have the right to walk away from harmful situations. And you have the right to say no to even the closest of friends or family members.

You have the right to choose what goes into your mouth, and you have the right to question the ingredients of unfamiliar food. You have the right to ask the waitperson to go back and get you more vegetables if you do not have enough. And you have the right to demand that your meal be prepared exactly as you need it to be. Most of all, you have the right to a life free from the obsession of food. You have the right to live free from the bonds of eating uncontrollably.

One of the most difficult situations I had to deal with during the early months of my recovery involved popcorn at the movies. My friend and I had decided to see a movie together, and he chose to have popcorn. While it wouldn't have been my first choice to sit next to him while he ate one of my most dangerous binge foods, I recognized that he had the right to eat whatever he wanted.

The problem came when he decided to explain in detail how delicious the popcorn tasted. My first reaction was to scream and yell at him, but I forced myself to remain calm and take a deep breath. After a minute or two, I looked him in the eye and asked him if he would tease an alcoholic in the same way if he were drinking beer. He looked shocked and replied, "Of course not." I then explained to him that teasing me with food was exactly the same.

To this day, my friend has never done anything like this again. He has remained one of my biggest supporters, even going out of his way to make sure I have the proper foods I need. Had I handled the situation differently, I may have lost a very valuable friend. His intentions weren't mean. He simply didn't understand the ramifications of what he was doing.

What if you are at a birthday party for your niece and your cousin keeps asking you if you want a piece of cake? He tells you that you have to eat cake to celebrate the child's birthday. After you have said no politely several times, he still continues to insist, waving the cake under your nose. The most important thing you need to do at that minute is get away from the cake. Gently push his hand away and walk into another room. The bathroom is always a good idea if you really need a few minutes to collect your thoughts.

When you have calmed down, maybe even meditated or said a prayer, then you can deal with your cousin. If you are absolutely too distraught and need to leave, offer a polite excuse and go. But if you are able to stay, find your cousin. Explain to him that you would appreciate it if he would not put food in your face. Tell him that you are on a strict food program after discovering your allergy to certain foods, cake being one of them. If you feel comfortable, explain the addictive nature of your disease with the comparison to alcoholism. If not, simply leave it at that—a food allergy.

In many cases, simply saying you have a food allergy or a medical condition will save you hours of lengthy explanations. The concept of addiction is difficult for many people to understand. You may also want to take it a step further by pointing out the seriousness of your affliction. Many food addicts we know tell people they will die if they eat sugar or flour. And considering the progressive nature of the disease, their explanation is accurate.

Whatever works for you, do it. But remember the rule used in one of the Twelve Step programs—"Say what you mean, mean what you say, but do not say it mean." In each of the examples mentioned, the key to expressing yourself was to remain calm and think about what you wanted to say before speaking. Damage done from words said in anger is often hard to repair. Why take the chance of alienating a good friend or concerned family member when it can be avoided?

Keep in mind that saying no to well-meaning friends or family members gets easier with practice. There will be times when you agree to something you wished you had not. Use those instances as lessons instead of punishments. Think about what you learned from the experience and how you can avoid similar occurrences in the future. Realize how it made you feel to do something you did not want to. And develop ways to say no next time you are asked.

If you are having an especially difficult time with saying no or are struggling with other hard-to-handle problems, you may want to seek professional help. The next chapter will discuss how to recognize when you need extra help. You will also find tips for discovering the right treatment method.

Read on and find additional ways to improve the quality of your life. And remember, you always have the right to say no. The choice is yours. No one else can make it for you.

14

I Need More Help

You have tried the food plan several times and you just cannot seem to go for long without eating your addictive substances. What should you do? Do you feel as if you want to give up? Continue reading this chapter to find out if you should seek some extra help with your program.

It is possible, even likely, that you simply need either a support group or individual counseling. You may be facing things that you cannot handle alone or haven't the experience to manage. If this is the case, you will want to take some time to research your options. In this chapter, you will learn how to tell when you really do need extra help and how to find the right counselor or program for you.

Roadblocks

First, let's examine several societal myths that may be holding you back from seeking treatment. Probably the biggest and most dangerous one of these is the idea that we should all be able to handle our problems alone. Most people who are trying to determine their emotional support needs struggle with this notion of self-sufficiency. Most of us were raised to be strong, not to cry when it hurts, and to protect the sanctity of our families. While all of these things seem honorable at first glance, it is important to look deeper.

Be Strong

Telling children or adults that they must be strong when tragedy strikes is asking them to ignore their natural need to experience the pain. It also adds to the hurt by attaching guilt. A person who has gone through a tragedy needs to experience the feelings that go along with the event. When we remind others to be strong, we are really telling them to deny their humanity. And at the same time we are placing guilt on them for something they cannot control—their feelings.

Don't Cry

Similarly, reminding children or adults not to cry when it hurts causes them to deny their feelings and feel guilty for their "weakness." Crying is a healing experience. Most people are unable to deal with the uncomfortableness of seeing another in pain, however. They will try to make the person feel something different. How many times have you seen someone offer a child a lollipop to stop crying? Or, what about those people who immediately offer an adult a cup of tea to stop the tears? Whatever the substance or activity, the message is the same—you should not cry.

What is wrong with crying? Why is it labeled as bad to do in public? It has to do with our pursuit of perfection in both our looks and behaviors. The Puritans and the Victorians both imposed harsh behavior rules on citizens, many of which involved outward appearance in public. While these attitudes have dissolved to some extent, in many cases substitutions have been created.

Overly emotional people were banished to their beds and labeled ill during the early 1800s. Today, we are encouraged to deal with our issues behind the closed doors of a therapy session and not in public. No matter what the time, the message is still similar—expressing feelings in front of others is not acceptable. But why? What would really happen if someone saw you cry? Would that make you any less of a person?

Though many of society's attitudes have grown more liberal

over the years, rules about emotional expression have changed little. A few years ago, an article praised Jacqueline Kennedy Onassis for her bravery during her husband's funeral. The article pointed out that not once did the public see the first lady cry as the president was put to his final resting place.

Sarah Ferguson and the late Princess Diana have been openly admonished in both the American and British press for showing even the slightest bit of emotion. Both women, during extremely difficult times in their lives, had broken down in public. Instead of seeing this as a normal reaction to extraordinarily painful circumstances, reports of nervous breakdowns followed each incident. In short, both the press and the public panicked when they saw royals crying.

With attitudes such as these, it is easy to see where you might get the idea that crying is wrong or bad. But, it is not. Crying allows you to release some of the pain you are feeling, which in turn helps you to begin healing. Sure, no one likes to cry, but sometimes, especially when dealing with the amount of changes you may be, it is necessary. By attaching shame to the action, you are only increasing your pain.

Protect the Family

Another harmful message we are given is to protect the sanctity of our families. How can this be negative? Shouldn't we protect our family members from harm? Of course. We are talking about protecting the "sanctity" of your family, not individual members. The best way to explain this is to use the title of a famous book by Claudia Black—*Don't Talk, Don't Trust, Don't Feel.* In her book, Black describes this as the message many addicted families were raised with.

Think about your own family. How many times were you instructed not to tell someone something or to pretend that things were different than they really were? If you grew up in an alcoholic family, for example, were you trained to cover for the alcoholic if he or she were drunk? Did you lie to others so they wouldn't know just how unhappy your family life was?

Were you always taught to pretend things were normal when company was present? Did you or your parents put on a "show" when others were there?

This is what is meant by the sanctity of the family—protecting the appearance of the unit. Unfortunately, this protection comes at the expense of individual members. For instance, think about the child who always lies to his father's employer to cover up a hangover. Through this behavior, he develops a pattern of ignoring his need for honesty. The child may have a strong need to discuss the situation or even to maintain his integrity by being honest. But these needs go unmet whenever the employer calls.

In extreme cases, protecting the sanctity of the family results in serious injury, even death. Newspapers and talk shows are filled with examples of abused children refusing to discuss their torture in the name of protecting the sanctity of their families. The reasons for this are many. A common explanation is that children are "supposed to" love their own flesh and blood, even if those family members are abusing them. In other words, the societal belief that you should not hate or harm your family members becomes the reason many do not seek extra help.

Putting the sanctity of the family before your own well-being will only keep you trapped in your pain. Contrary to what you may believe, there is no honor or pride in protecting people who have caused you pain. Your own mental and physical health should be your primary concern. Your family members are adults who are capable of taking care of themselves. Your responsibility is to yourself and your needs. And if one of your needs is to have professional or group counseling, then you must listen to your desire.

Do You Need Extra Help?

How do you know when you need extra help? Following are some questions to ask yourself when trying to decide. It is important that you answer them as accurately as possible. Don't worry what your answers mean; just write what you feel. It is a good idea to give yourself a few minutes with each question. Your first reaction may be an automatic no due to your denial mechanism.

Answer yes or no to the following questions.

1. After being abstinent from your addictive substances for at least two months, do your emotions still feel out of control?

2. Even though you have given it a serious attempt at least six times, are you still unable to remain abstinent consistently?

3. Do you still feel deeply depressed each day, the only difference being that you are not eating your addictive foods anymore?

4. Are you experiencing suicidal thoughts even though you are not eating your addictive substances?

5. Have you tried to share your feelings with others but found them unable to understand what you are experiencing?

6. Is there a secret you have carried around with you for years that is weighing heavily on you?

7. Does your life seem to be unstructured or unmanageable?

8. Are you unable to do much of anything because you are paralyzed by fear?

9. Do you seem to argue constantly with the people in your life, often becoming involved in heated incidents?

10. Does it seem impossible for you to abstain from your addictive foods?

11. Have you wanted desperately to share your feelings with someone but could not find anyone willing to listen?

12. Are you living with an addict who is actively using his or her substances?

13. Since you made some changes in your life, are you having an extremely difficult time adjusting?

14. Do you feel you can no longer continue to live your life the way you have been?

15. Are you desperate to change your situation but seem unable to do so?

16. Does your life feel completely overwhelming?

17. Is there a great deal of stress in your life?

18. Has something tragic happened that you have been unable to deal with?

19. Do you feel completely powerless to change your life?

20. Are you ready and willing to share your problems with someone else?

If you have more than five yes answers, you may want to consider seeking outside help. Keep in mind that this quiz is not intended, nor should it be used, to measure the success of your recovery from food addiction. Fewer than five yes answers does not in any way mean that your program is successful. It is simply an indication that you may not need additional help. Similarly, more than five yes answers does not mean your program is not solid, only that you may need some extra support.

> When I was experiencing an enormous amount of stress and unhappiness in my life from my job situation a few years ago, I found that my recovery program from food addiction was as strong as ever. Though I was in an incredible amount of pain, I was still doing the same things I always had. I continued to weigh and measure my food, talk about my feelings, and stay in touch with my higher power.
>
> Even though most times I didn't feel like working my program, I did it anyway. If I really got into trouble, I prayed for the willingness to do what needed to be done, and it was always there. When I least feel like taking care of myself, that's when I most need to take action. The strength or success of my program is measured by my willingness to do whatever it takes to avoid my addictive substances. It is not determined by the events in my life.

Many food addicts report having little or no difficulty avoiding their problem foods during major tragedies. Their problems come when things are going wonderfully, as they are uncomfortable with experiencing these foreign feelings. Either way, this quiz will not determine how effectively you are working your program. Only an honest evaluation of your life can inform you of that.

If you have decided you require additional help, how do you go about finding exactly what you need? Where do you start and what if you do not have any money or insurance to help?

Overeaters Anonymous

The best place to begin is at a Twelve Step meeting such as Overeaters Anonymous (OA). These meetings are filled with other people who are struggling to develop healthy relationships with food. There are no professional counselors at the meetings, and attendance is free. The benefits of attending meetings with others experiencing similar incidents are many. The camaraderie, understanding, success stories, and even the pain of members will provide you with a chance to relate to others in ways not usually possible with nonfood addicts.

Though meetings in each area may differ in format, the premise for all is the same. Individuals interested in developing healthy relationships with food come together to share their experience, strength, and hope about recovery. Usually, you will find OA meetings in church basements, Sunday school rooms, community centers, or even senior centers. They are anywhere a large group of people can gather for an affordable price. Even though many meetings are held in churches or synagogues, the groups are not affiliated with any religious organization, political movement, or ideology.

So, how do you find OA meetings in your area? The easiest way is to call Information or look in the white pages of your phone book for an Overeaters Anonymous listing. The number given will direct you to a recorded message of times and locations of OA meetings. Or, you will be given the telephone numbers of several members who will share meeting information with you personally.

If your area does not have such a listing, you can do several things. First, you can dial Information and simply ask for a listing for Overeaters Anonymous without providing a city or town. This will help you to find the meeting nearest to you. Additionally, you can check out the national Web site at http://www.overeatersanonymous.org. Or, you can send a letter to OA's World Headquarters: Overeaters Anonymous, Inc., 6075 Zenith Court Northeast, Rio Rancho, NM 87174-4020. Finally, you can call for information about meetings in your area at (505) 891-2664.

What can you expect at these meetings? Usually, there will be a discussion about anything from dealing with holiday problems to feelings to the Twelve Steps of the program. Think of it as a group of friends who get together in an organized way to discuss life's problems. Before attending a meeting, however, keep a few things in mind.

Overeaters Anonymous does not allow "crosstalk," meaning that you may not interrupt the speaker. You must wait your turn. Also, advice-giving is discouraged. In other words, if you are sure you have the answer to someone's problems, it is suggested that you do not share it during the meeting. It is also a good idea to concentrate on your own problems and not try to fix others. These rules allow members to openly share feelings and thoughts without fear of criticism. The meetings are designed to promote honest sharing.

During OA meetings, you will hear talk about a higher power, perhaps even God. It is important to remember that, though it may seem to be at first, OA is not a religious program but a spiritual one. It is not necessary to believe in God to successfully work the program. Many atheists and agnostics have found recovery through OA. The only requirement is to remain open to spiritual growth and tolerant of others' beliefs.

Finally, you may feel uncomfortable at first because of the intense level of honesty at many meetings. If this is so, remember what you have learned about the importance of sharing your feelings and the healing value of crying. While not all meetings are filled with emotional sharing, if you do encounter one, try to think of it as a healthy exchange of feelings.

As you know, a symptom of the disease of food addiction is isolation. Breaking through the isolation and shame of food addiction is one of the first steps to recovery. This makes OA meetings invaluable to those seeking change in their lives. Group members who share their feelings are actually helping to heal their pain.

If you really do not like the first OA meeting you attend, try another. Some meetings may just not be right for you or may be going through a rough time at the moment. The "flavor" of any meeting changes often, sometimes even weekly. So, either give the meeting you attended another shot or look for another one.

In most areas, OA meetings are held at least three or four times a week, some having more than triple that. It is suggested that you try six meetings before deciding whether or not the program is right for you. Attending this many meetings prevents you from making rash decisions or allowing your denial mechanism to guide you.

If OA does not seem right for you, or even if it does and you need extra help, you may want to consider individual counseling. With the emotional difficulties that today's complex world presents, the counseling options available to you are many. The yellow pages are filled with names of counselors, even listing their primary areas of specialization.

Choosing a Counselor

What should you look for in a counselor? You will want to think first about the characteristics of a counselor that are important to you. Ideally, you will want to find someone with whom you feel comfortable discussing your deepest problems. The following questions will help you get a better idea of what you should look for in a counselor. On some of the questions, you may not have a preference at all—this is fine.

1. Do you feel more comfortable sharing your feelings with a man or a woman?

2. What's the approximate age you are looking for in a counselor? For example, if your counselor were twice as old as you, will it feel too much like a parent-child relationship?

3. What general philosophy do you need in a counselor? (For example, is it important for you to find a counselor with experience and belief in addictions treatment?)

4. What about location? Should your counselor be close to work so you can run over during your lunch hour or nearer to your home for evening or weekend visits?

5. Are there certain hours you need your counselor to be available? Do you have small children who make it impossible to get away during the day? Is your work schedule too demanding for weeknights? Whatever your needs, finding someone who supports them is essential.

6. Is the counselor affiliated with support groups should you want to become involved in one?

7. Do you prefer a counselor in private practice or one affiliated with a larger counseling center?

8. If you do decide to stay in OA, does the counselor support this method of treatment?

9. What are the fees and what portion will your health care insurance cover?

10. If finances are a problem, is the counselor willing to discuss a payment plan? Does the counselor work on a "sliding scale" fee—when counseling fees are adjusted to your income level?

11. In case of severe emotional problems, does the counselor work with a licensed psychiatrist or psychologist?

12. What type of professional qualifications do you need in a counselor? For example, will you only consider a licensed psychologist or is someone with a masters in social work (MSW) acceptable?

13. Does the counselor belong to any professional organizations or attend seminars that would make him or her aware of the latest treatment options?
14. In the event of an emergency, can the counselor be reached after office hours or at home?
15. How long has the counselor been in the area? If it is only a short amount of time, why did he or she relocate?

Again, these questions are designed to help you select a counselor; they are not an absolute method of determining anyone's credibility. While it is not necessary to find answers to all of these questions, you will want to discuss the ones most important to you. Having such a list of criteria will help you when sifting through the pages and pages of listings in the phone book.

When you have found two or three counselors who you feel may be helpful to you, arrange an interview. Remember, a counselor is working for you, not vice versa. The only way to tell how comfortable you will be with a counselor is to sit down and talk with this person. And do not be afraid to ask questions during your interview. It is the only way you will find out what you need to know.

If this is your first experience with counseling, how will you know who is best for you if you only meet one person? It is like making a big purchase. You do not settle on the first car you test drive, so why should you settle on the first counselor you interview?

This brings us to another point—do not be afraid to say no to any counselor with whom you feel uncomfortable. When interviewing counselors, it is best to listen to your instincts. Even if you cannot put your finger on it, if something does not feel quite right, go to another counselor. All the while try to balance your feelings with your denial mechanism, which will be fighting your efforts.

The question, then, to ask yourself is this: is it me or the counselor? If you have interviewed several counselors and had the same feelings about all of them, you may want to rethink your motives. Are these things, for example, simply nitpicky problems that will not affect your treatment? If so, you may be unconsciously sabotaging your recovery so that you can return to eating the foods you love. If not, and the problems will truly interfere with your treatment, keep searching until you find the right counselor for you.

Choosing a Group

If you prefer not to attend individual counseling, why not try a private support group? Many counselors or counseling centers offer weekly support groups designed to help recovering people deal with their difficulties. This is usually an effective way to discuss your problems in a group setting if you want that option but do not feel comfortable in Twelve Step meetings.

When choosing a group, however, be careful to find out more information about it before agreeing to join. The following questions can help you develop your own list of criteria for a support group.

1. How many people are in the group and where in their recovery are they? For example, a group where everyone is in long-term recovery may prove frustrating. It may be difficult for you to discuss your problems if you are new to recovery.

2. What are the qualifications of the group leader? Beware of someone without any professional experience, as there are many money-making schemes in the world that can prove dangerous to you and your recovery.

3. Who are the other people in the group? Are they all males or females?

4. When and where does the group meet? Is it a place where privacy is possible or are there a lot of distractions?

5. Is it possible for you to attend one group meeting before making a final decision?

6. Can you be assured that your issues and identity will remain confidential?

7. If need be, is it possible to contact group members in between meetings?

8. How long have the current members of the group been together? You may feel like an outsider with a group of people who have been together for an extended amount of time.

9. Are there any people in the group who are overweight or struggling with eating or food issues?

10. Does anyone in the group have a physical addiction to a substance, food or otherwise?

11. What other issues are group members dealing with?

12. What are the "rules" of the group? For instance, is it okay for members to interrupt each other?

13. How long does the group session run, and, if it is only a short period of time, is there another group you can attend?

14. Do you need to attend individual counseling in conjunction with group meetings? Are there any other such requirements?

15. Will your insurance cover this group session or can you work out a payment plan if necessary?

These questions will help guide you in your search for a group in which you will feel comfortable. Again, it is important to research your options. If you try a group and do not like it, then find another one. All the while keep in mind your inborn resistance to recovery. And, remember, attending group meetings may not always feel good. In many cases, you will feel uncomfortable—this is often the case when we are growing the most.

If you have tried all or one of the previously mentioned methods and nothing seems to be working, you may consider inpatient food-addiction treatment. Similar to those for alcoholics, food-addiction treatment centers are a relatively new concept, quite different from the traditional "fat farms." In the past, many food addicts were sent away to camps or spas to lose weight by starvation and compulsive exercising. Today, however, food-addiction treatment centers have been created to deal with both the physical and emotional aspects of the disease. They provide inpatient, and in some cases outpatient, help for those unable to deal with the disease in an unstructured environment. Think of these centers as hospitals for people too sick to be treated at home. If you had diabetes, for example, there might come a point in your treatment when you would need to be hospitalized for a period of time. It is the same with food addiction.

> As an alumnus of one, I speak from experience when I say that food addiction treatment centers can save your life—the center I attended saved mine. I was too deep into my disease to even get myself to any kind of support group meetings, and individual counseling did not seem to be enough for me to stop eating. After some research, I found the structure and discipline I needed to begin my recovery program during a six-week stay. I truly believe that nothing else could have helped me like this.

Food-Addiction Treatment Centers

What can you expect at a food-addiction treatment center? Most include individual and group counseling sessions, nutritional classes, recreation therapy, and family treatment conducted in a communal setting with other food addicts. Somewhat similar to other treatment methods, these centers offer the addict a chance to develop a healthy routine that can be used long after treatment is completed.

How do you find a food-addiction treatment center? Here is the contact information for two centers that treat food addiction:

> Turning Point of Tampa, 5439 Beaumont Center Boulevard, Suite 1010, Tampa, FL 33634; (800) 397-3006; Web site: http://www.tptampa.com

> The Willough at Naples, 9001 Tamiami Trail East, Naples, FL 33962; (800) 722-0100; Web site: http://www.thewillough.com

These are intended as a guide to help you get started looking for a center that can best serve your needs. It is not a comprehensive directory of those places subscribing to the sugar- and flour-free method of treatment. Because individual needs vary, you will need to contact the treatment centers you are considering attending. You can also look in your local phone book. Treatment centers are usually listed under marriage, family, child, and individual counseling. Or, try asking a counselor or doctor to recommend additional food-addiction treatment centers.

One of the newest trends in food-addiction treatment is the development of weeklong inpatient programs. Created to provide services for those who don't need hospitalization or direct medical support, these workshops are affordable to individuals. Ranging in price from $700 to $1,500, these programs are offered nationwide. Here is one such program:

ACORN Food Dependency Recovery Services,
    P.O. Box 2218, Orland Park, IL 60462; (708) 226-1858;
    Web site: http://www.foodaddiction.com

Choosing a Food-Addiction Center

No matter where you find a center, you will want to investigate the treatment methods used, as well as the qualifications and reputation of the institution. Following are some questions you may want to ask before making a final decision.

1. What kind of professional qualifications does the center have? For example, is it a licensed psychiatric facility?
2. Is the treatment center dedicated solely to addictive disorders or is it part of a medical hospital?
3. Will they send you free information about the center?
4. How long is the average stay at the center?
5. What are the qualifications of treatment personnel?
6. Is individual as well as group therapy provided and how often?
7. What is the treatment center's philosophy?
8. Does the center support a sugar- and flour-free method of eating?

9. Are meals weighed and measured?

10. Is dietary counseling available with a licensed dietitian who is aware of the physical aspects of food addiction?

11. Are support or self-help groups part of the center's treatment process?

12. If needed, is it possible to involve your family in treatment?

13. What is the success rate of patients after leaving the center?

14. What type of support is offered upon leaving the facility?

15. Will your insurance cover the expense and, if not, can a payment plan be negotiated?

16. Is the facility geared toward anorexic or bulimic patients only?

17. What type of people are in treatment? For example, are there many overweight people? How many males and females?

18. Will your specific medical needs be supported during your stay? If you have a knee problem, for instance, will you be excused from difficult activities?

19. What portion of the treatment is dedicated to exercise?

20. How are meals structured? Do you eat with others or alone in your room?

Only you can determine which of these questions you will want to ask when considering a treatment center. You may find it necessary to have additional information as well. Do not be afraid to thoroughly investigate any center you are considering, as that is your right. Also, beware of facilities with a high ratio of exercise. You may find yourself at a health spa instead of a food-addiction treatment center.

When investigating treatment center options, ideally you will want to find a place that offers both individual and group counseling on a regular basis. Interaction with others at mealtime is also vital. And it is important to find a facility that provides additional help after you leave treatment. Some centers, for example, offer weekend programs around the country for former patients or weeklong stays at the institution for those experiencing problems. Such options will be invaluable as you progress in your recovery.

So, if you have decided on a food-addiction treatment center as your only hope of recovery, it is vital that you choose carefully. As with anything, find out all of the necessary information. Ask if you can have the names and numbers of former patients willing to speak with you; then make an informed decision based on the choices open to you.

Now, you have discovered the options available to you when you need extra help. And you have the tools needed to find what will be most effective for you. It may take some time to discover the method of treatment that is exactly right for you, but if you are persistent, you will find what you need. And remember, ultimately you are the only one who should decide what to do. That is your right.

In the next chapter you will learn about another important method of treatment to be used in conjunction with your food plan. It is something we all dread but that has incredible benefits. With it, you can permanently change your life for the better.

15

You Want Me to What?

Now that your curiosity about this method of improving your recovery is piqued, it is time to introduce you to a concept you may have forgotten about—exercising. We know. We know. We can hear your protests already. Before you dismiss the notion, read this chapter and discover a new way of looking at exercise.

Exercising

If you are like most food addicts, you have tried many exercise programs. You may have even invested large amounts of money in state-of-the-art equipment or health spa memberships only to give up almost as quickly as you began. Why is that? And why can't you seem to exercise on a consistent basis?

Well, you will be happy to know that one of the major reasons for your exercising difficulties is your food addiction. With all of the energy it took to combat a disease you did not even know you had, who could think about exercise? In most cases, your life was so centered around food that there was little time for anything else. And the last thing you wanted to do was something so strenuous and taxing on your overweight body. It is difficult enough for a normal-sized person to remain committed to an exercise program. For someone overweight, underweight, or obsessed with food it is nearly impossible.

Think about how hard it is to even walk when you are overweight; imagine how difficult it would be to do anything even slightly more strenuous. Couple this physical difficulty with the tension and stress of being in public and it is no wonder exercising can be a tragic experience for many food addicts. But once you have taken steps to get into a recovery program, your exercising attempts will be as different as the rest of your life.

If you have experienced any episodes of abstinence from your addictive substances, then you already realize how different this change can make you feel. Instead of the foggy, drugged feeling you were once a slave to, you now have clarity of thought and an incredible amount of energy. Your outlook on life has probably changed, and you awaken each morning with a zest for life instead of the dread you used to feel. With all of these positive changes in your life, doesn't it make sense that your attitude and experience with exercising will be different too?

If you have yet to attain abstinence from your addictive substance, your attitude about exercise may still have changed. Just the fact that you are working to improve the quality of your life means you are on the way to experiencing success. This is indicated by your willingness to read this far.

Remember, if you work at it, you will begin to see concrete results. And one of the ways to do this is to begin exercising regularly, no matter what the state of your food program. If you have been unable to abstain from your addictive foods up to this point, a sensible exercise program may be just what you need. It may push you over the line to success. So, read on and find out where to start.

The most important thing to do when beginning an exercise program is to check with your doctor to determine your physical limitations. You have already spent so many years hurting yourself, do you really want to continue? Make this book the first step you take in being kind to yourself on a regular basis. Continue the pattern by contacting your physician.

After checking with your doctor, your next step is to find a regular time each day when you can exercise. Before you panic, realize that you will only need to actually exercise three or four times a week, not every day. If you are convinced that you have no time in your busy schedule to exercise, think twice about your conclusion. Remember when we discussed ways in which you can make extra time for your program earlier in the book? Well, now is the time to put those methods into practice. Think about the activities in your life that are no longer serving you well. Just the fact that you have stopped bingeing should give you some extra time, since it used to take up much of your day. Take some of the time you used to spend bingeing or thinking about eating and turn it into your exercise period.

There Are Lots of Options

When determining an appropriate time, keep in mind your personal preferences. For instance, are you the type of person who prefers to exercise first thing in the morning? Or would you rather do your exercising in the afternoon or evening? Whenever it is, choose your time to coincide with your preference.

If you are unsure exactly what time you want to pick, then pay attention to your natural rhythm during the day. Do you, for example, seem to be most active when you first wake up, or is it in the evening when you hit your peak? A little self-knowledge will go a long way when determining your ideal exercising time.

Choose an activity that you really enjoy. It does not necessarily have to be fitness-oriented. If you love to shop, begin walking around a mall in the early morning or late evening hours. Be careful, however, not to stop and browse too many times, as you will not get the full benefits of exercise.

Do you have a passion for looking at old houses? If so, then tailor your exercise program to include walking around the historic section of your town or city. Or maybe it is the beach or beautiful foliage that you adore. If so, incorporate these into your exercise program. A walk on the beach or through the woods three times a week will do wonders for your recovery program and for your physical condition. Whatever it is you love, add it to your exercise program and have fun!

When deciding the type of exercise you will do, it's important to choose an activity that you want to do. Do not start jogging, for example, just because someone told you that you should. That only makes sense, right? Yes, but it certainly needs repeating since so many food addicts have long lists of reasons why they shouldn't do something.

Are there activities that you would never even consider doing? Or is there something you have always wanted to try but never have because of the limitations you have placed on yourself. For instance, have you always wanted to try roller-skating or bowling? If you are like most food addicts, you have a long list of "shouldn'ts" where exercise is concerned. The only way to rid yourself of them is to examine your beliefs regarding exercise. What do you think will happen if you start exercising? What do you fear?

To discover your reasons for resisting activity, make a list of everything that comes to mind when you think about exercising. Write down all of the things you believe will take place if you actually begin exercising. After you have done that, carefully examine your list. Are any of these things valid reasons for not exercising? Be rigorously honest when answering this question.

Contrary to what you may believe, most food addicts do not avoid exercise because they are lazy. Instead, it is fear that prevents them from actually exercising. How many times have you been ready to exercise when you were crippled with fear about what other people would think? Did you actually go through with exercising, or did you head straight for the refrigerator to soothe your fear?

> For me, it was a crippling fear that someone would physically hurt me if I went for a walk. That, coupled with the physical pain of actually moving 328 pounds of flesh, kept me a prisoner in my own home. I was desperately afraid of someone sticking a knife in my back as I walked down the street; therefore, I avoided going out in public. I would never have even considered putting myself through the torture of dealing with this fear for the mere sake of exercising. The sad part is that the only place I was actually in danger of getting hurt was in my mind.

Can you relate to this? Do you have similar fears? Are there reasons why you are sure it would be too painful to exercise? Is your life filled with limitations similar to the ones described? Do you spend most of your time avoiding activities?

If so, write down those things you fear and look at them. How realistic are they? What are the chances that the thing you fear most will actually happen?

While some of your fears about exercising may be perfectly valid, most are concoctions of your mind. They prevent you from doing healthy things for yourself. If you do, however, suffer from a recurring, paralyzing fear that you cannot deal with yourself, you may want to seek professional help.

All or Nothing

Still another reason many food addicts resist exercising is due to an "all-or-nothing" attitude. How did you feel, for example, when we mentioned walking as a good way to exercise? Did it seem like a "wimpy" activity instead of "real" exercise such as jogging? If you said yes, then you may be suffering from the all-or-nothing attitude that plagues most food addicts.

Before we explain it to you, first think about how many exercising machines you have purchased over the years. How much did they cost? How long did you actually use them? Where are they now? By examining your answers to these questions, you will begin to see what we mean by all-or-nothing.

For most addicts of any kind, it is difficult to grasp the concept of moderation. Addicts either throw themselves 150 percent into an activity or refuse to participate, making it impossible for them to put forth moderate amounts of energy. While at first glance this may seem a very admirable trait, think about the burnout rate. After a few weeks of giving 150 percent, what's left? A pile of broken promises is usually the result, thus the all-or-nothing attitude.

Addicts, due to the excessive nature of their diseases, are usually unable to find the middle ground in their activities. This is especially true of food addicts who begin starvation diets only to end up bingeing on everything in sight a few days later. That's why, as with many other aspects of your recovery program, it will be necessary to change the way you view exercising.

It is not required, not even recommended, that you run out and do three hours of exercise a day as part of your recovery program. Thirty minutes, three times a week is all that will be needed. Did you hear that? Thirty minutes, three times a week, not three hours a day. And you do not need to invest one cent in any kind of exercising equipment. The best kind of exercise you can do does not require any investment of money on your part. You need only walk out your front door.

You don't think taking a brisk walk is that effective? Forty to fifty minutes of walking gives you the same results as twenty to thirty minutes of jogging. And in your case, especially if it is been a long time since you have done any type of exercise, it is a good idea to start slowly. Work your way up to a faster pace, though jogging is not necessary and may even be painful if you have knee or other medical problems.

So, why are you waiting? Put on your sneakers and walk around your neighborhood for thirty minutes. While you are doing so, notice all of the things you miss when speeding by in your car. Are the flowers just beginning to bloom, or do the changing leaves look beautiful? Is the freshly fallen snow pretty, or does the deep green grass seem especially nice today? Whatever it is, notice it as you walk, and before you know it your thirty minutes will be over.

As you walked, did you feel some negative messages run through your head? Were you more critical of yourself than usual as you walked? Did it seem as if those painful thoughts you have worked so hard to release all came flooding back at once? If so, there is a reason for that.

Body Image

Your pain may be due to your beliefs and thoughts about your body image. Most food addicts are dissatisfied and constantly overconcerned with their body shape and weight, which results in a negative body image. Having a negative body image, in turn, may lower your self-esteem and keep your food addiction active; it may even prevent you from taking part in some social situations.

Think about all of the activities you avoid due to your body size. This may be true even if you are not overweight. When is the last time you went swimming? bowling? skiing? It is not necessary to do these activities in order to have healthy feelings about your body. Avoiding activities you enjoy, however, is a sure indicator of a negative body image.

What exactly is a body image? Your body image is the thoughts and feelings you have about the way you look; it consists of two parts—the physical and the psychological. The physical aspect of your body image concerns a given body feature or movement. And the psychological aspect reflects your feelings, thoughts, or beliefs about your body.

The enormous number of "props" humans possess makes it possible to hide the psychological aspects of body image. For example, have you ever seen someone who is perfectly dressed? Did you just naturally assume that this person had positive beliefs about his or her body? It may seem that way to you, but in many cases perfect clothing is used to hide feelings of dissatisfaction and unhappiness with the body's image.

The problems most food addicts have with their body image revolve around three specific external body perceptions.

Physiological Aspects

First, the physiological aspect includes the way your brain detects weight, shape, size, and form. If your brain is not able to determine correct measurements, you may have an unrealistic picture of what your own body looks like.

Take a handful of marbles (or rocks) and estimate how much you think it weighs. Then, put it on a scale to find out exactly how many pounds it is. Were you close? Now, try the same thing with a bowl of water. Pour some water in a bowl and estimate how many ounces it is. Did you guess right? No matter how you did with this exercise, the point is still the same. As a food addict, you likely have a hard time determining the actual measurements of items. As previous chapters have discussed, you can see where this will be dangerous when determining your food portions.

If you are unable to determine proper measurements, where does that leave you with your body size? Do you really know what you look like? Is the image you have of yourself consistent with that of your actual weight?

The best way to determine how accurate your concepts are is to find someone who weighs about what you do and take a good look at that person's body. This exercise takes some tact, however. If you are unwilling to ask someone to help you, then look at people in magazines or on television. Use diet advertisements that show before and after pictures. Keep in mind that television adds at least ten pounds to a person's appearance. Or ask a close friend or your spouse how much he or she weighs and work from there. You may be surprised at what you find. But keep in mind that weight looks different on each person.

Conceptual Aspects

The second perception that gives most food addicts difficulty is the conceptual aspect, or mental picture, they have of their bodies. How do you see yourself? What is the image you carry around in your mind of your body, and how accurate is it? Many food addicts view themselves as being either much larger or much smaller than they actually are. Few have accurate pictures of their body sizes.

How can you deal with this problem? The best, and sometimes most painful, way is to take a tape measure and find out exactly what size various parts of your body are. Measure your chest, waist, hips, calves, arms, ankles, and wrists; then write down what each one is. Take some string and measure out the corresponding amount for each part of your body. Then, tape or glue each piece in the shape of a circle to a piece of paper.

When you are finished, look at the actual size of your body parts. Are they what you expected? Did the actual ones come close to the picture you had in your mind? No matter what your perceptions were, now you have a realistic idea of your body size. This knowledge will enable you to work on learning to accept those body parts with which you are unhappy. You may want to save your measurements to compare them to where you are in a few months. The results might surprise you.

Psychological Aspects

The last body perception most food addicts struggle with is the psychological, or emotional, aspect of their body images. This includes the way you feel about your body. Do you hate the way you look? Is it hard for you to even look in a mirror? Do you detest dressing up or shopping for clothes?

A yes answer to any of these questions may signal a problem with the way you feel about your body. You can further determine any difficulties you may have. Write down all of the thoughts and feelings that come up when you think about looking at yourself in the mirror. Are most of them negative? Do you have many more unkind thoughts than kind ones? If so, you are not alone. Most food addicts report experiencing self-loathing and revulsion about their bodies.

So, what can you do to change your thoughts and perceptions about your body? Several of the techniques already discussed can be extremely helpful in changing your body image. Using affirmations to counteract the negative messages will help, as will visualizing yourself having positive feelings about your body. (See chapter 10 to review these tools.)

Other things you can do include treating your body with kindness and respect even if you don't yet feel that way. Change your hair or clothing style. Discard loose-fitting clothing. Tuck in your shirt. Take a bubble bath. Use body lotion. Wear nice perfume. Or smile at yourself in the mirror. Refuse to hurt your body anymore. Be gentle with yourself. Put rubber gloves on when you wash dishes. Get a manicure, a massage, or a facial. It doesn't matter what it is as long as it's something nice for your body.

When you have begun to feel better about your body, exercising will become more natural and thus easier for you. So, if you find yourself unable to exercise on a regular basis, then begin working on your body image. Before you know it, if you are persistent, you will be exercising regularly. The following are some additional tips to keep you moving.

1. Set a regular time each day to exercise and stick to it as you would any other appointment in your life.

2. If possible, find someone else with whom to exercise. Knowing another person will be there may help to motivate you.

3. Throw an "active" party where attendees play badminton, volleyball, basketball, or some other group sport.

4. Reward yourself—not with food—after you have done your exercise. If you have walked a half hour, for instance, allow yourself time to play solitaire if that is what you love to do.

5. Do a variety of exercises to prevent boredom. Take a walk one week, then try roller-skating, or whatever else you like, the next.

6. Find activities that don't feel like exercise. If you love to dance, for example, try taking a class. The key here is to fool yourself into exercising.

7. Remind yourself that exercise does not take away your time. Instead, it creates more of it by giving you increased energy and stamina to pursue those activities you love.

8. If you are having trouble finding time to exercise, get up a little earlier in the morning. It's a great way to start your day out right. If you are not an early bird, use your lunch hour—provided you can find time to still eat your meal—for a midday pick-me-up.

9. Try using one- or two-pound weights when exercising to increase the benefits of your workouts. This is especially helpful for those with tight time schedules, as it maximizes the benefits from exercising.

10. Be persistent. Remember that the first few weeks are the hardest, so hang in there and know that it will get easier.

11. Chart your progress. If you are weight lifting, measure yourself once a month. Or, if you are walking, see how much farther you go during your thirty minutes. A record of your accomplishments will help spur you on during those hard-to-get-started times.

12. Remind yourself of the psychological benefits of exercising. Not only are you helping your body to be more physically fit, but you are also increasing your self-esteem and helping to manage the stress in your life.

13. Do something else while you are exercising. If you ride a stationary bike, watch television or listen to the radio to make the time go faster. If you love to talk, invite a friend to join you on your walk to help make it more enjoyable.

14. Create a "Fitness Contract" with family members or friends who share your desire to exercise. If you commit to each other the amount and type of exercise you will do, it will be harder to back out or find excuses.

15. Incorporate exercising into volunteer work. If you have always wanted to help others, find a way to do so while exercising. Maybe there is a daycare center nearby that needs someone to help with recess. Or perhaps a homeless shelter in the area needs someone to load or unload food. Whatever it is, be creative and you will reap the benefits of a well-rounded exercise program.

These are only a few suggestions to help you in developing and continuing an exercise program. It is not necessary, and perhaps even impossible, to use them all. As with everything in this book, find what works for you and stay with it. If you have tried three or four activities and none seem to be quite right, try more until you find the one you like.

When designing your exercise program, remember to put any perfectionism you may have aside. Remind yourself regularly that there is no perfect exercise program. Perfectionism will only cause frustration. Remember the all-or-nothing attitude we discussed? The results of perfectionism are similar.

Both will ultimately cause you to abandon your exercise program altogether.

At first, for example, you may be able to walk for only twenty minutes at a time. While your first reaction may be to criticize yourself, think, first, about how many minutes you exercised a month ago. None, right? Isn't twenty minutes a major accomplishment over your previous record? Think about it. You have increased your exercising program twenty times more than before! That is the kind of result for which most stock traders would kill!

However you design your exercise program, remember that you are worth the effort and time put into it. You deserve to feel better about yourself. And more important, it is your right to work at having a healthy body. So, why are you waiting? Go ahead! Exercise your right to a healthy, happy new life.

In the next chapter, you will read about ways to manage your food plan during holidays and special occasions. Read on and further increase your chances of recovering!

16

Do I Get a Day Off?

So, what about vacations, holidays, and special occasions? Are you supposed to remain abstinent even during these difficult times or do you get a day off? Considering everything you have learned, what do you think the answer is? By this point, you already know a lot about food addiction. You are aware of your own personal addictive foods. And you even know a good amount about developing a healthy lifestyle. Yet, dealing with holidays or special events may still be tricky for you.

Staying on Track during the Holidays

In this chapter, you will learn how to remain abstinent from your addictive foods through holidays and other tricky situations. Tips on managing your recovery program during these times and special activities you can do to make the days easier will also be provided. Read on and discover how to stay in recovery year-round.

To begin, let's examine the attitudes surrounding these special events that can cause problems for many food addicts. Special occasions are viewed by most people, including those with normal eating habits, as times to "go wild" eating whatever they want. These times are seen as rewards for eating healthy during the year. Luscious food is looked at as the ultimate way of celebrating.

Let's take Christmas as an example. Beginning at least two months before the big event, magazines and newspapers offer recipes and tips for making the perfect holiday meal. On television, we are shown warm and loving holiday family scenes. All of these include the "perfect" foods—cookies, pies, cakes, bread, and so on—used to show our families how much we love them.

Store shelves are overflowing with edible treats, from tinfoil-wrapped chocolate Santas to imported caviar. Individuals are urged to show their loved ones how much they care by splurging on these special foods. And for those with little time, malls and grocery stores alike offer gift baskets and stockings containing everything from exotic cakes to smoked beef. These specially made showpieces are portrayed as perfect gifts for the ones who have everything.

As if this isn't hard enough, we face the additional stress and pressure of increased responsibilities during this time. We are expected to buy, wrap, and give gifts to our loved ones as well as gather with them to feast on our favorite foods. For those with dysfunctional families, the holiday season may mean spending time with people who have harmed or abused them. Additionally, we are supposed to decorate our homes and participate in special community or church holiday events.

Then, of course, there are the Christmas cards to write and the holiday parties to attend. The charity drives and food gifts to collect for the needy. The visits with Santa and trips to the movies for special holiday showings. On top of all of this, we are expected to continue performing well at our jobs. And, in many cases, we need to increase our productivity to deal with greater workloads. Exhausted yet?

Can you see why Christmas and other special occasions can be dangerous times for a food addict? Think about your own life. How many of your holiday memories involve food? What is it you most look forward to about special events? Is it the wonderful food that you know will be in abundance, or is it the fact that no one will say anything if you eat it? Do you see these occasions as times to "pig out" without feeling remorse?

If you answered yes to most of these questions, what does that leave you with now that you have decided to remain abstinent from your addictive substances? That is a question only you can answer after you have done some thinking. This is the first step to changing your attitude about holidays and special occasions. Instead of looking at these times as an excuse to binge, figure out what each event means to you personally.

For example, if you have always looked forward to the special kosher foods at Hanukkah, think about what the celebration means in your life today. Can you look at this holiday as a time of dedicating yourself even more to your religious convictions? Or can you use it to share your strength and commitment with others?

If it's the turkey you drool over at Thanksgiving, can you view the holiday as a special time to share with your friends and family? As a time of being grateful for all of the gifts you have been given? Instead of anticipating the Easter chocolate, find spiritual meaning in the holiday. Think about how grateful you are for the life you have been given. Have fun hiding eggs for the children—the plastic kind, not the edible ones.

Whatever the holiday is, find special meaning in it for yourself. It doesn't matter if others do not share your new attitude about holidays. In many cases they will not. What is important is that you can see the difference. You deserve to enjoy each and every holiday and special occasion. Just because you are abstinent from your addictive substances does not mean you can't enjoy yourself. It is simply a matter of having fun in a different way.

Making It Easier

Before we discuss how to change the way you have fun at holiday time, read about some special activities you can do to make it easier. This way you can come through the event without bingeing. First, do not project or obsess about what could or may happen. Remember the slogan "One day at a time"? Well, use it to keep focused on the present. Despite appearances, nearly all holidays and special events last only twenty-four hours, not two months as advertisers would have you believe. So remain centered in the present moment.

If you are at work, for example, you do not need to obsess about the New Year's Eve party in four weeks. Simply concentrate on whatever you are doing at that minute. This will help lessen the anxiety you feel about the event. As you have already learned, events created in your mind are usually more dangerous and stressful than they are in reality. By focusing on the present, you will avoid building a wall of fear in your mind, thus lessening your stress level.

Next, break tasks down into small parts instead of doing everything at once. The quickest way to build up resentment and stress is to wait until the last minute to do your holiday chores. These are the feelings that will cause a food addict to find solace in food. So, instead of waiting until the last minute, plan ahead. If you have an unusually large Christmas card list, for example, begin writing out ten cards a night starting the day after Thanksgiving. This way the task won't seem so overwhelming.

If Thanksgiving is at your house this year and the cleaning seems overwhelming, vow to do one room each day beginning the week before the event. This will help you avoid feeling bogged down with cleaning and cooking at the same time. Another good idea is to start cooking the foods that will stay fresh at the beginning of the week. With this system, you will not become overwhelmed by last-minute tasks.

Additionally, operate under the motto "If in doubt, leave it out" when making holiday plans. In the previous example, for instance, if you do not feel comfortable cooking an entire Thanksgiving meal, then don't. Make other arrangements. If someone else will not cook, then make reservations at a restaurant you know will accommodate your food needs. If you do not feel comfortable attending the office holiday party, then avoid it or leave early.

Determining what events you will or will not attend takes a good deal of honesty on your part. While in some situations you may clearly see the danger to your program, others may not be so obvious. For this reason, it is necessary to evaluate each event carefully before attending. If your office is holding a

Fourth of July barbecue and picnics are dangerous for you, then don't go. If you have convinced yourself that you must attend to keep your position, you may be using this as an excuse to eat.

Remember, there is no holiday function or special event that you must attend. Your life or death is not dependent on being present at these occasions, and that includes your livelihood. Would you expect a person with the flu to attend?

Discovering Dangerous Situations

So, how do you know if a situation has the potential to be dangerous to your recovery program? The best and most effective way is to look at your thoughts and feelings about the event. Are you anticipating having an awful time, or do you feel extremely nervous whenever the subject arises? Do your palms get sweaty at the mere thought of entering the room where the event is taking place?

What about your physical condition? Are you suffering from ailments usually associated with stress? Do you, for instance have an upset stomach or diarrhea? If so, you may want to avoid the event or, at the very least, make arrangements to protect yourself.

> For me, it was my first Thanksgiving that caused extreme concern. Having been in recovery for only four months, I was terrified at the thought of facing the biggest eating day of the year. I had visions of bingeing on those special foods I loved so much and losing the most precious thing in my life—my recovery. I didn't want to go back to the overwhelming pain I had faced. I also didn't know how I would react when faced with plates full of luscious treats.
>
> For a few days before, I suffered from severe diarrhea and was in a constant state of nervousness each time I thought about facing the day. Attending my support group and reading daily did not seem to curtail the horrible anticipation I felt about the holiday. Each time the subject came up, I was afraid and pessimistic. I was unable to even believe that I would come through the holiday with my recovery program intact.

I began to practice the things I knew worked—concentrating on how far I had come, writing about my feelings, and praying. Soon, an idea came into my mind. I decided to ask for one room in the house—the event was to be held at my parents' home—that did not contain any food. I knew it would be unfair to expect other members of my family to avoid eating things I chose not to eat. But asking them to refrain from bringing food into one room seemed like a reasonable request.

It worked so well that I continued the practice for several more years. For the holidays that were not at my parents' house, I simply did not go into the room containing all of the desserts. Or, if it got too much for me to take, I left. Many times going for a walk or to the bathroom has saved me from potentially dangerous situations.

This brings us to yet another activity you can do if things get too difficult—leave or take special precautions. If you have your heart set on attending an event that you think may cause problems, then plan to stay only for a short amount of time. Make arrangements to do something with a friend at a designated time that will force you to leave early. Or, if it is easier for you, arrive after the meal has been served. Be careful, of course, not to come in the middle of dessert.

Bringing Your Own Food

Another solution to tricky situations is to bring your own food. If you are committed to weighing or measuring your food but do not feel comfortable doing it in front of others, prepare it at home and bring it. Don't worry what others will think. If they do not like it, simply leave. In most cases, however, a short explanation about your medical problems will do wonders to create an environment of understanding.

This advice also holds true for restaurants. If the party you are dying to attend, for instance, is at a pizza parlor or fast-food restaurant where you know you cannot get the food you need, bring your own. Most places—unless, of course, they are kosher—will be understanding, even helpful about letting you eat your food with their other paying customers. In some cases, you may be asked to pay a "plate charge" or fee for taking up space in the establishment. Look at this as a small price to pay for enjoying the event. If you weren't in recovery, the food you ate would have cost a lot more than the small amount the restaurant is charging. Wouldn't it?

Also, don't be afraid to call ahead to restaurants to find out what they will be serving. In some cases, it may be possible to have your meal weighed and measured for you in advance, if you feel comfortable with that arrangement. The point here is that if you do not ask, no one is going to know what you need.

> At my sister's wedding, for example, I spoke with the caterer of the reception to arrange to have exactly the foods I needed. Though I was nervous, as maid of honor, I sat at the head table and weighed and measured my food just as I would have if I had been home. While I previously had visions of everyone staring at me, I soon found that almost everyone was too preoccupied with their own meals. No one even looked at what I was doing with mine. It was a wonderful learning experience for me to realize that my cup and scale didn't stand out as much as I thought they would.

Persistance is another key to making special occasions easier. If you are having trouble arranging for the food you need at the event you are planning to attend, then think of another way. Be persistent and you will find a method for getting exactly what you need. There is always a way, if you hang in there. If you are staying with someone who does not have the kind of food you eat, consider going to the supermarket or bringing your own. You may even want to offer to cook the evening meal. This will allow you to prepare exactly what you need.

With the introduction of salad bars and prepackaged produce in grocery stores, the food you need is only a short drive away. If you get stuck, buy a premade salad, small can of tuna in water, and can of corn or chickpeas for your dinner. You may also want to purchase dressing or spices to add some flavor, but it is not necessary in an emergency. For lunch, just add a fruit. And with breakfast you can simply go to the produce, dairy, and cereal aisles to get what you need.

Sticking to your meal plan is the same as taking medicine when you are sick. Your food is your medicine. And you must be persistent, even creative, when finding ways to get what you need to make and keep yourself healthy.

Alternate Plans

Similarly, having an alternate plan will help you remain abstinent during special events. What will happen if you go over to your friend's house for a Valentine's Day party and she forgot to buy the food you need? What will you do? Or what if the restaurant cooks your vegetables in butter? Then what? If you are prepared, neither situation will be a problem for you.

Keep an emergency bag in your car for such unexpected problems. If you have chosen to follow the recommended food plan outlined in chapter 11, then get two large cans of vegetables, a smaller can of a starch, a small can of a protein substance, a cup, scale, measuring spoons, fork, and can opener and put them in a bag in your car. The trunk is best so you will not constantly see it.

> I have mushrooms, beans, corn, and tuna in my car. With this bag, I am set for anything. No matter where I am, I always have exactly the type of food I need. And it sure has come in handy. Just the other day, I forgot my measuring cup and had to use the one in my car. This bag has saved my program on more than a few occasions.

One last thing you can do to make holidays easier is to invite someone who is following the same plan you are to the celebration. If you are in a support group, ask one of its members to help you get through the occasion by being there. You may want to have someone there during the preparations, which can be a dangerous situation. If you volunteered to make a food you do not eat, for example, ask for company when shopping or preparing the food. If cleaning up the kitchen is hard, then ask for help with that. Whatever it is you need, ask for it.

Note that someone who is understanding of your disease, though not necessarily affected by it, can be just as helpful as someone who is following your food plan. The important thing is to have someone with you.

> My family has always been extremely supportive and helpful of my efforts, though they do not follow my food plan. My first few holidays in recovery I was unable to be around the food at cleanup time. I found myself resentful at every uneaten bite on other people's plates. When I didn't participate in the cleanup, no one even mentioned my absence. Additionally, family members have always been willing to discuss menus ahead of time, even preparing special foods for me. All I have to do is ask.

Creating New Activities

Now it is time to learn about different ways of having fun during special events and holidays. A major part of recovery from food addiction involves developing new behaviors. This means that instead of using eating as your main entertainment at holiday gatherings, you will need to create new activities to amuse yourself.

For instance, have you ever thought of taking a walk or playing a game? Do you love the outdoors? Then, gather as many people as you can for a nature walk or if you are up to it, a game of hide-and-seek. If you prefer more relaxing activities, then try chess, checkers, or Monopoly. Or how about renting a video or going to a movie?

If you are the creative type, try organizing a craft activity. If it's near Christmas, make tree ornaments or pot holders to be used as gifts. Sew a pillow or knit booties for the new baby in the family. Begin crocheting a blanket for yourself or make a patchwork quilt with everyone creating a few squares. Whatever it is you love, do it. The items you make will serve as nice reminders of your first efforts at developing healthy new holiday traditions.

What if you are having trouble finding a new activity? The best way to discover one is to walk through the aisles of a toy store. Examine the items that interest you. Is this something you could bring to family gatherings? If not, is there a "grown-up" equivalent? When doing this, be sure to look in the game aisle, as there will be many items for adults. But, remember, if you see something you really want, don't limit yourself because you are afraid it is not "adult" enough. Try not to worry what others will think. If you are interested in it, then have fun doing it!

You can also take some of the things you have learned in recovery and elaborate on them. For example, has writing really helped you through many rough spots? Then create the beginning of a short story and have everyone else write a paragraph or two to complete it. Or, if you have found a really profound piece of writing that has helped you and it is appropriate, share it with others. Be careful, however, not to overwhelm those in your life with too much information at once.

If the hardest part of holiday gatherings is being cooped up in the house with everyone, then create an outside activity. At Christmas, for example, ride around and look at how beautifully the houses are decorated. Thanksgiving is a good time to attend a football game. A walk on the beach is perfect during the Fourth of July holiday. Be creative and you will find exactly the activity you need to help safeguard your recovery.

Also, if you are too overwhelmed or upset by the occasion, attend a support group meeting, if possible. If you have been attending Overeaters Anonymous meetings, find out if there is a gathering on the holiday. We know many food addicts who regularly attend Thanksgiving Day meetings.

If there is not a meeting available, consider starting one or try attending another Twelve Step support group. Alcoholics Anonymous, for example, has round-the-clock meetings during Christmas and New Year's Day in many areas of the country. While some meetings labeled "closed" are open only to alcoholics, anyone is welcome at "open" meetings. Remember, your disease is the same as an alcoholic's, only the substance you use is different. Whatever effort is required to make it through the holiday or special occasion will be worth it when the day is over.

Learning to Cope

As one food addict in recovery for several years points out, "Halloween, Thanksgiving, and the December holidays were always binge times—and miserable times—when I was actively in the disease, and they were difficult, slippery times in early recovery. [After] seven years with a steady day-to-day abstinence and lots of recovery for which I'm grateful, I still need to take special precautions."

This food addict notes that when he first entered recovery, he stayed away from situations if he sensed they might be a problem. "My first six months in recovery, I did not go to restaurants at all, turned down invitations to parties, went to an Overeaters Anonymous meeting on Halloween night, visited my parents at times other than meals, and left the office Christmas party early."

After several months in recovery, he began to feel more comfortable attending gatherings. "As I began to have enough recovery to attend social functions with food, I learned to prepare in ways that 'normal eaters' do not. I called ahead to the host of a Super Bowl party and said I needed to eat only at mealtime, was bringing my own food, and might have to leave if things got too difficult regarding the food. I also asked the waiter at restaurants for food without my addictive substances—and when I was not sure I was understood, I brought out the 'alternative food' I had packed; when my family or work responsibilities included socializing with food, I often offered to have the affair at my house or to be actively involved in the planning so I was sure to be able to get my needs met."

Today, this food addict is happily in recovery and enjoying life at a normal weight, free from food cravings. "This program works when I work it," he said. "There are still times I choose not to be in social situations at holidays where there is lots of food. Is that extreme? To a 'normal eater' it often seems so, even to me when I am back in denial or wanting to be a 'normal eater' myself. But I am not, and I have things to do today that keep me out of bingeing. When it works, do not fix it."

While his precautions may seem overwhelming to you, realize two things. First, everyone's recovery is different. You may not need to take all of these precautions to remain abstinent from your addictive substances, but then again, you may. Only time and honesty will tell. When a situation arises, you will know what you need to make it through.

If your actions seem "extreme" to others, remember that they are not in your situation. Your main concern should be to stay away from substances that have caused you pain in the past. How could someone who has not experienced your level of devastation due to these foods understand why you are doing what you are to avoid your addictive substances?

Second, no one is telling you that you must avoid social functions. You have the right to choose not to go anywhere if you feel it will threaten or harm your program. *You are not required to stay home,* nor is it necessary, in order to work a successful program. Your recovery from food addiction is about making healthy choices that will enable you to live a fuller, happier life free from food cravings. It is not about becoming a hermit.

A Higher Quality of Life

The quality of your life will improve dramatically as you enter and stay in recovery from food addiction. You will no longer "lose" hours of your day to bingeing in secret, ashamed of your actions. It will not be necessary for you to spend hours, even days, planning your binges only to be left feeling frustrated after eating more than you imagined possible. But most important, you will never need to call yourself "bad" for the things you have eaten if you are following your food plan. Aren't these rewards worth taking a few extra precautions?

Should you "slip" or binge during a holiday or special occasion, keep in mind that it does not have to turn into a relapse. If you have eaten something not on your food plan, then stop with that. You do not have to continue eating. You can get right back on your food plan. Don't wait until tomorrow or Monday. You have the right to begin your recovery program again immediately.

Also, remember that you are not a failure, only a human being. There is no such thing as perfection in any area of life. So, give yourself a break and begin again immediately. The longer you wait, the harder it will be to become abstinent. And you are certainly worthy of the best possible life you can make for yourself. You deserve to live free from the obsession of food. It is your right and your responsibility. No one else can do it for you. You must make a conscious choice to recover. This includes holidays and special occasions.

So, read on and finish the book. Remember, no matter what happens during a holiday or special event, you are worthy of living an exceptional life without bingeing. You deserve it and you must take responsibility to make it so. The choice is yours and the time has come to make a decision. Only you can decide. What is your choice?

17

Choices and Chances

Before you read about how to improve the quality of your life
in this chapter, we want to take a minute to congratulate you
for getting this far. Do you realize that you have just about finished this book? That, by itself, signifies your desire to recover
from the disease of food addiction. Give yourself some credit.

How did it feel to give yourself credit? Was it uncomfortable, or did you decide not to do it? Whether or not you actually went through with it, your reaction shows a lot about your
self-esteem. Did you congratulate yourself but refuse to really
feel the pride of your accomplishment? Or didn't you even acknowledge what you have done? If you did either one, you probably suffer from low self-esteem, which is common among food
addicts.

Self-Esteem

Because of the commonness of low self-esteem, this chapter is
dedicated, in part, to the topic of self-esteem. As a food addict,
you have experienced a devastating loss of self-esteem. Prior to
reading this book, and perhaps even still, you believed that
your food problem was solely your fault. You thought you
could control it if only you were a better person. And you believed that because you could not control it, you were a bad
person worthy of all sorts of punishment.

With all of these negative perceptions, where does that leave
your self-esteem? Do you see yourself as someone who doesn't

really deserve happiness even though you desperately strive for it? Is your worth measured in the number of things you do for others? Or do you keep yourself so busy that you don't even have time to be alone? Is it painful to imagine spending an evening by yourself without eating?

If so, it is important for you to continue reading this chapter to find out how to further improve your life by raising your self-esteem. Contrary to what you may think, your self-esteem is not a frivolous concept worthy of little or no attention. Your feelings about yourself determine the choices you make in your life. These include decisions involving your career, spouse, family relationships, financial standing, and education level. Knowing this, does self-esteem sound like something you don't need to pay much attention to?

Here are some quick and easy tips on how to raise your self-esteem. Most of the suggestions take only a few minutes a day, so you have no excuse not to use them.

Say "I Love You" to Yourself Every Day

You are what you think. When you tell yourself that you are worthless or no good, you become just that. It's a self-fulfilling prophesy. If you think bad, negative thoughts about yourself, you will attract negative things that act out those beliefs. Many of us grew up believing it was not acceptable to love ourselves, that people would not like us if we did. We thought we would be considered conceited, but that is not true.

People are attracted to those who have a high opinion of themselves—not arrogant, vain, stuck-up people, but individuals who respect themselves. If you cannot yet fully respect yourself for your personal characteristics and traits, start by realizing what a miracle your body is. Without any thinking on your part, your body automatically breathes and digests. That alone deserves your respect.

Every day, as often as possible, say to yourself, "I love you." In the morning when you are brushing your teeth, look in the mirror into your eyes and say, "I love you." On the way to work, instead of obsessing about the day ahead and what needs to be done, think to yourself or say out loud, "I love you." You don't have to believe it, just say it. You will be amazed at the difference in your life after you have done this for several days. You will start to believe you are worthy of good things happening—that you deserve them. Your life will change for the better. When you begin to love yourself, you will look at life differently. You will not be willing to settle for second best.

You will also realize that you have a right to make your dreams come true. And you will begin to take steps toward achieving them. It will not happen overnight, but it will happen. It may be a little hard at first, but it will be worth it when you begin to see the results. How hard can it be to say three little words to yourself each day? Go ahead, give it a try!

Change What You Tell Yourself

As we discussed in chapter 10, an affirmation is a statement, negative or positive, that reflects how you feel or want to feel about yourself. Most of us have used affirmations all our lives, unfortunately not the kind that promote high self-esteem. Negative affirmations eat away at your self-esteem, making you believe you are unworthy, fat, incapable, ugly, old—the list is endless.

While it is easy to spot these blatant negative affirmations, others are more subtle and harder to notice. But they are just as dangerous to your self-esteem—maybe even more so because they reflect deep-rooted, unconscious beliefs you have about yourself. Thoughts such as "I'm just lucky, that is why I got the promotion; there was no one else to give it to" and "If they really knew me, they wouldn't like me" are negative affirmations in disguise. By saying these things to yourself—and reinforcing the belief that you are not good enough—you are making them a reality in your life.

In the same way, when you say positive affirmations to yourself, you are increasing your self-esteem. You are working toward raising your opinion of yourself by changing your thoughts. The more often you say positive affirmations, the more you will begin to believe them. And your whole life will change.

Your affirmations should be positive, present-tense statements, usually action-oriented. For example, say, "I am attractive," instead of, "I am becoming attractive." Writing your affirmations makes them even more powerful. Take ten minutes in the morning or at lunch to write down your positive thoughts. Some changes will come quicker than others, but if you are persistent, they will come.

Forgive Yourself for Your Mistakes

No one is perfect. We all make mistakes, sometimes big ones. This is what makes us human. Who among us is not ashamed or regretful of something from the past? Today, we are different people. You most likely have learned from your mistakes. You needed these experiences to be the person you are today. Now it is time to let go of them.

Many people use their past mistakes to punish themselves, which results in low self-esteem. How many times have you used excuses like these to prevent yourself from being happy: "I am a bad person because I stole a candy bar when I was twelve years old" or "I am a dishonest person because I cheated on my math test in eighth grade"?

When you beat yourself up like this, you are destroying your self-esteem. It becomes a vicious cycle. You punish yourself about things you cannot change, which makes you hate yourself even more. The good news is that you can break the cycle. It does not have to be like this.

Remind yourself that making mistakes, no matter how severe you think they are, does not mean you are a bad person. Some of your mistakes may seem more serious than the previous examples, but the solution is still the same. Accept that no matter how hard you try, *the past cannot be changed.* And you do not have to continue to pay for it with guilt either. Forgive yourself and watch your self-esteem soar!

Live for Today—Stay in the Present

"I will be happy when _____"—you fill in the blank. How many times have you said these words: "I will be happy when I lose weight"; "I will be happy when I get a new job"; "I will be happy when I get married"? These, and thousands of other such statements, postpone your happiness, which lowers your self-esteem. You are telling yourself that you don't deserve to be happy until a certain event happens. What you are really saying is that you aren't good enough right now, today, to be happy. And when the long-awaited event does occur, there will always be another and another. This makes it impossible for you to ever achieve happiness and high self-esteem unless you begin to accept yourself today.

Making outer conditions responsible for your happiness puts you on a roller coaster of emotions. If you feel good only when things go your way, you are left miserable a great deal of the time. As long as your happiness is tied into the achievement of future goals, you will never be satisfied. You will always need more to be happy. And if you need more, then you are telling yourself that you are not good enough. This damages your self-esteem.

While goals, dreams, wishes, and fantasies play a necessary part in your life, even adding to your self-esteem, it is important that you live for right now. You are perfect just as you are at this very moment. Sure, there are things you would like to work on, but you are still a worthwhile, beautiful person just as you are today.

Right now, make a list of five positive characteristics or traits about yourself. Whatever it is, write it down. Keep this list in a safe place and refer to it when you start thinking of all the things you don't have. Give yourself permission to be happy and have high self-esteem *today*.

Stop Comparing Yourself to Others

You are unique and special. There is no other person exactly like you in this world. You may have things in common with others. But no one has all the traits, characteristics, dreams, hopes, and wishes that you do. You see and do things exactly like no other human being. Therefore, how can you even begin to compare yourself to another? It's like comparing apples to oranges. Each is unique and luscious in its own way, but not for the same reasons.

When you compare yourself to others, you lower your self-esteem by not accepting who you are. Each time you make a comparison, you say to yourself, "I am not good enough. I need to be more." This prohibits you from recognizing your value.

Instead of admiring a famous actress, model, or sports figure, realize that both of you are people. Neither of you is perfect, but each has wonderful parts that make up a unique person. The only difference between the two of you is that the other person has high self-esteem, which contributes to a successful, positive self-image.

It is what you say to yourself, therefore, that makes the difference. If you continually look at how short you fall of being a perfect person, you are damaging your self-esteem. Improving yourself can be a helpful and positive experience. It is important, however, to remember that you are perfect just the way you are, with or without the goal for which you are striving.

Remember that just because someone else's life looks perfect doesn't mean it is. Everyone has problems.

Listen to Your Inner Feelings

You have an inner voice that guides you, telling you your feelings and needs. Yet, many people ignore it, working hard to live up to others' expectations instead. When someone else tells you how you "should" act, what you "should" want, or how you "should" behave, they are hurting your self-esteem. Though it may not be done intentionally, it still harms you.

Since each person is unique, no one else can determine another person's needs. Not everyone's standards are the same—nor should they be. No matter how close you are to someone, there is always a side you keep hidden. This makes it impossible for anyone to make fully informed choices or decisions for you.

Many times low self-esteem is the result of trying to live up to someone else's expectations while ignoring your own. Some believe it is easier to do what others want than to live with the guilt of disappointing or angering someone, especially in the case of parents. But when you do things you don't want to, you trap your true self. And usually you don't do a good job, which lowers your self-esteem even further. While it may seem easier at the time to do as someone else wishes, in the long run the damage you do to your self-esteem isn't worth it.

So, go ahead, be true to yourself, no matter how impossible you may think your dream is. Don't you at least owe it to yourself and your self-esteem to go after it?

Set Your Boundaries and Be Firm

"No" is a complete sentence. Learn how to say it. Setting your boundaries—deciding what you will or will not accept—is an important part of achieving high self-esteem. You give yourself the message that what you think and feel isn't important when you let others take advantage of you.

Placing others' needs or wants before your own lowers your self-esteem. When you do this, you tell yourself that other people are more important than you are. Of course, there are times when everyone does things out of obligation. It's when those times become the rule rather than the exception that your self-esteem is diminished.

Wanting approval from others is healthy. It is unhealthy, however, when approval-seeking turns into a need rather than a want. When you need approval, you become willing to do anything for it, thus crippling yourself to act except when others agree. Stop trying to please others.

Take Proper Care of Yourself

When you take care of yourself by eating right, exercising, and getting enough sleep, you're telling yourself that you are special. You are proving that you deserve to be taken care of and that you are worthy of good care.

Too many times you may get so busy taking care of others

that you forget about yourself. Your parents, friends, spouse, children, even pets, come before you do. With so many people in your life, it can be easy to forget about yourself, but you deserve care too.

When you don't take care of yourself, you feel bad about yourself. Lack of sleep makes life seem depressing and not enough exercise makes you feel lethargic. You have a choice.

Do Something Nice for Yourself

Show yourself how special you are by doing something nice for yourself each day. If your first thought after reading this is "I don't have time," then you had better think again. Doing something nice for yourself can take as little as one second.

Look in the mirror and say, "I love you. You are great!" That is something nice, and it only took five seconds—ten if you speak slowly. If you have more time, take a long, hot bubble bath by candlelight while you listen to relaxing music.

Do you have a hobby? Make time for it. Show yourself how important you are. Take a walk, meet with a friend. Sit quietly for a few minutes or meditate. Sing! Dance! Write! Blow bubbles! The list is endless! It doesn't matter what the activity—or nonactivity—is, as long as you enjoy it. Go ahead, have fun, and increase your self-esteem!

Follow Your Dreams

Everyone has a dream. What's yours? Have you always dreamed of performing on Broadway, writing the "Great American Novel," or traveling to Alaska? Whatever it is, make plans to do it! You are worthy of having your dreams come true.

Set daily goals to make your dreams a reality. If you want to write a novel, spend fifteen minutes each day writing. You don't have to write the whole thing in one day. Do a little at a time, and your dream will become reality. Setting and working toward your goal allows you to achieve your dreams, which increases good feelings about yourself. And nothing compares to the feeling of getting where you want to go.

Don't Put Yourself Down, Even Jokingly

Sure everyone loves a clown, except the clown. Making a joke at your own expense may get you laughs, but it will not increase your self-esteem. Saying mean things about yourself, no matter how funny they may be, affects your self-esteem. As with affirmations, after a while you begin to believe them.

Putting yourself down diminishes the good feelings you have worked so hard to attain. Is a moment of laughter worth that? There are too many naturally humorous things in life about which you can joke. Do not use yourself as a target. While everyone else is laughing, your self-esteem is crying out in pain.

This does not mean that you should stop laughing. Laughter is good for your self-esteem and you should enjoy life, but not at your own expense. You have worked too hard to sabotage yourself now.

Surround Yourself with Positive People

Did you ever notice that there's always one in every crowd—the first one to criticize good things or find the negative in an otherwise positive situation? The only way to handle this type of person is to get as far away as possible! If you are like most people, you have enough negative thoughts about yourself without any additional help. You don't need negative people in your life. And you have a right to protect yourself from them by staying away.

Negative people are toxic to your self-esteem. At first, you may not notice the damage done to your positive feelings about yourself, but it is there. Little by little, the negativity eats away at your self-esteem. If the negative person is someone who cannot be avoided, then work extra hard at filling yourself with positive messages. As Eleanor Roosevelt pointed out, "No one can make you feel inferior without your consent."

Stop Blaming Yourself

How many times have you taken to heart something that has nothing to do with you? Just because the store clerk treats you rudely does not mean you are a bad person. It means he or she is having a difficult day or has other problems that have nothing to do with you. Many of us take things like this personally. As one woman put it, "I used to blame myself when it rained." This may seem silly to you at first, but consider all of the things you take personally that are beyond your control.

It's not your fault the traffic is heavy and as a result you're late. You cannot control your boss's character. The day would not have been any better if you had worn your blue shoes instead of your black ones. Chances are that your husband wouldn't have remembered your anniversary if you had been different.

All of these situations, and many more, are absolutely beyond your control, and taking responsibility for them only decreases your self-esteem. You have no control over other people's actions. They are individuals capable of and responsible for their own actions. You are a wonderful person just as you are and, unfortunately, bad things still happen.

Continue Your Education

For many, the word "education" conjures up thoughts of wicked teachers and boring work, but it doesn't have to be that way. Learning can be as easy as reading the paper once a week or looking at a magazine about your favorite hobby. When you acquire knowledge, you grow, which naturally increases your self-esteem.

Think you don't have anything worth learning about in your life? How about being a better parent? spouse? friend? lover? employee? Bookstore and library shelves abound with sources of information you can use to further your education.

Do not stop there! What about attending a seminar or a night class? One-day, inexpensive personal-growth seminars are currently being offered across the country. You can learn everything from how to improve your grammar to how to deal with stress. These seminars give attendees simple, effective, easy-to-use suggestions in a short amount of time.

For more information about seminars in your area contact CareerTrack and Fred Pryor Seminars at 1-800-334-6780 or 1-800-255-6139; SkillPath, Inc. at 1-800-873-7545; or Hazelden at 1-800-328-9000. Go ahead! Attend one! You are worth it!

If you're looking for more in-depth information, consider attending a local university. Most colleges offer noncredit, continuing education classes at greatly reduced rates. For a little more money, you can work toward a degree in something you have always wanted to know more about. Contact your local university for more information, and watch your self-esteem rise!

Why not take that exercise class you have been avoiding? Learn about aerobics or weight training. Dance or craft classes are only a phone call away. Whatever it is, learn more about it and you will feel great about yourself.

Refuse to Believe in Failure

Before she died in 1906, Susan B. Anthony, who spent her life fighting for women's voting rights, gave us this message: "Failure is impossible." Read this over and over again. Commit it to memory. You cannot fail. "Failure is impossible."

Webster's New World College Dictionary, second edition, defines failure as "a falling short, a losing of power or strength, a not succeeding in doing or becoming." These are all arbitrary judgments. Who decides when you have failed? Is it written somewhere? Does a big red sign with the word "failure" on it come down from the heavens? Of course not. That would be silly, but isn't labeling yourself a failure based on nonstandardized criteria just as silly? Many Twelve Step programs operate under the theory that there are no failures, only slow successes. Just because things aren't going your way doesn't mean you have failed. The only time you have failed is when you believe you have. The choice is yours!

Be Responsible—Keep Your Word

Yeah, it is a cold, rainy Monday, and when 7 A.M. rolls around, the last thing you want to do is get up for work. Why should you? You work hard. You deserve some time off, right?

Maybe, but consider the price. When we fail to meet our responsibilities, we feel guilty, thus decreasing our self-esteem. Sure it is nice to have a break. Everyone needs that. But it's important to do it in a responsible, fair way in order to keep your self-esteem intact. If you really need a day off, try to arrange something with your boss. You may be surprised by his or her understanding.

Honoring your commitments is important in all areas of your life, not just work. Think about how you feel when someone lets you down. It hurts, doesn't it? It may even cause some problems or inconveniences in your life. Remember when the baby-sitter didn't show up the night you had two tickets to the hottest show in town? Or what about the time your co-worker failed to provide you with the necessary information for your report, causing you to work until midnight?

While it is important to note that failing to meet your commitments affects other people, the most dangerous damage it does is to your self-esteem. The guilt you feel over these incidents lingers, eating away at the good feelings you have worked so hard to establish. People who honor their commitments and behave responsibly increase their self-esteem with each act.

Of course, there will be times when it is impossible to meet every commitment you have made. In those times, an honest explanation of the situation should be sufficient, but first be sure you are really unable to keep your word. Not wanting to do something isn't always enough of a reason. Think of the temporary discomfort as the road to high self-esteem.

Invest in Yourself

Make a commitment to yourself. You are worth it! You deserve it. Set aside some time each day, or even each week if that is the most you can manage, to follow the suggestions we've just discussed. That is the only way they will work. Don't say you cannot spare fifteen minutes a day for something as important as this.

You will get out of them exactly what you put into using them. If you are consistent and work hard, your self-esteem will soar. What better investment is there?

As you probably noticed, the preceding tips have little or nothing to do with food, but instead with life. There is a reason for that. When you have figured out how to work your food plan and avoid your addictive substances, you begin to learn about living a life in which food is not the entire focus. These tips, then, are a reflection of the growth you will experience as your recovery progresses. Take the ones that work for you and leave the rest. If you have tried the first three but don't seem comfortable with them, go on to a few more. And keep going until you find the ones that are effective for you. But be sure to give it at least two weeks before deciding you don't like a particular suggestion. This will allow you enough time to experience any results. You may have to look carefully, though, when only using them for such a short amount of time.

Whatever method you decide to use to improve your self-esteem, remember that by reading this book you have already changed your feelings about yourself. Now, you know that it is not your fault you are fat. You have a disease. The same way some people get cancer, you got food addiction. Your food cravings and lack of self-esteem are symptoms of your disease, not moral reflections of your character.

But unlike someone with cancer, you have a choice about whether or not you recover from your disease. You can follow the suggestions in this book, refrain from eating your addictive substances, and work at recovering on a regular basis. Or you can choose to put this book away and never deal with your addiction. Either way, there is no shame in your choice, only repercussions from your decision. But shame does not have to be involved, as you have the right to make whatever choice you want.

If you choose recovery, your life will not always be perfect, but it will be one hundred times better. And based on many food addicts' experiences, this is a low estimate. You will no longer be driven to eat certain foods. Your head will be clear, and you will be alert to life's possibilities. Instead of feeling desperate and alone, you will realize that no matter what happens around you, you can have hope. You will know that very few negative things are ever permanent. And you will learn to respect yourself and others, allowing the space needed for growth.

No matter what you choose, now that you have read this book, your life will never quite be the same. You know too much to return to eating the way you have in the past. Even if you continue to eat the same amount, somewhere in the back of your mind you know that this book is there for you. You are aware that unless you change your eating patterns, the quality of your life will not improve.

It is up to you. As always, the choice is yours: an exciting, wonderful, new life free from food cravings or the life you have now. It doesn't seem like much of a decision, does it? May you find the path to recovery and the strength to heal from your food addiction.

Notes

Chapter 1: First, the Facts

1. *Alcoholics Anonymous,* 3d ed. (New York: Alcoholics Anonymous World Services, 1976), xxviii.

2. David B. Herzog, M.D., and Paul M. Copeland, M.D., "Medical Progress: Eating Disorders," *The New England Journal of Medicine* 313 (1985): 299.

3. Glenbeigh Health Sources of Tampa, *The Glenbeigh Guide to Eating Disorders/Food Addiction and Food-Related Problems* (Tampa, Fla.: Glenbeigh Health Sources of Tampa, n.d.), n.p.; Anne Katherine, *Anatomy of a Food Addiction: The Brain Chemistry of Overeating* (New York: Fireside/Parkside, 1991), 18.

4. Michael A. Schmidt, *Childhood Ear Infections*, The Family Health Series (Berkeley, Calif.: North Atlantic Books Homeopathic Educational Services, 1990), 18.

5. Andrew Weil, M.D., and Winifred Rosen, *Chocolate to Morphine: Understanding Mind-Active Drugs* (Boston: Houghton Mifflin Company, 1983), 9.

6. Schmidt, *Childhood Ear Infections,* 62.

7. Zoe S. Warwick et al., "Taste and Smell Sensations Enhance the Satiating Effect of Both a High-Carbohydrate and a High-Fat Meal in Humans," *Physiology and Behavior* 53 (1993): 561–62.

8. Robert Lefever, M.D., and Marie Shafe, "Brain Chemistry: Combinations of Foods in the Blood Trigger Effects Very Similar to Alcohol," *Employee Assistance* 3, no. 8 (March 1991): n.p.

9. Ibid.

10. Katherine, *Anatomy of a Food Addiction,* 17.

11. Kenneth Silverman et al., "Withdrawal Syndrome after the Double-Blind Cessation of Caffeine Consumption," *The New England Journal of Medicine* 327 (1992): 1109.

12. Ibid.

13. Lefever and Shafe, "Brain Chemistry."

14. Schmidt, *Childhood Ear Infections,* 87.

Chapter 2: The Research

1. Kenneth G. Goodrick and John P. Foreyt, "The Business of Weight Loss: Why Treatments for Obesity Don't Last," *Journal of the American Dietetic Association* 91 (1991): 1245.

2. "Losing Weight: What Works. What Doesn't," *Consumer Reports,* June 1993, 348–49.

3. Ibid., 349.

4. Ibid.

5. Jane E. Brody, "For Most Trying to Lose Weight, Dieting Only Makes Things Worse," *The New York Times*, 23 November 1992, A12L.

6. Ibid.

7. Bob Hill, "A Weighty Solution: Tom Wadden Puts a Lift into Weight Loss," *Syracuse University Magazine*, June 1993, 38.

8. Allan S. Kaplan and D. Blake Woodside, "Biological Aspects of Anorexia Nervosa and Bulimia Nervosa," *Journal of Consulting and Clinical Psychology* 55 (1987): 649–50.

9. Steven Lally, "Sweet Relief with On-the-Spot Tranquilizers," *Prevention*, September 1988, 30.

10. David B. Herzog, M.D., and Paul M. Copeland, M.D., "Medical Progress: Eating Disorders," *The New England Journal of Medicine* 313 (1985): 299.

11. Philip A. Horrigan, *The New Challenge of Chemistry* (n.p.: Marshland Publishing Company, 1985), 288.

12. Lally, "Sweet Relief," 30.

13. Samuel Homola, *Secrets of Naturally Youthful Health and Vitality* (New York: Parker Publishing Company, Inc., 1971), 48.

14. Ibid.

15. Ibid.

16. J. Fuller and G. Jacoby, "Central and Sensory Control of Food Intake in Genetically Obese Mice," *American Journal of Physiology* 183 (1955): 279–83; R. Nisbett, "Taste Deprivation and Weight Determinants of Eating Behavior," *Journal of Personal and Sociological Psychology* 10 (1968): 107–16; J. Rodin, "Effects of Obesity and Set Point on Taste Responsiveness and Food Intake in Humans," *Journal of Comparative Physiology and Psychology* 89 (1975): 1003–9.

17. J. A. Grinker, J. Hirsch, and D. Smith, "Taste Sensitivity and Susceptibility to External Influence in Obese and Normal Weight Subjects," *Journal of Personality, Sociology and Psychology* 22 (1972): 320–25.

18. Peter J. Rogers and John E. Blundell, "Separating the Actions of Sweetness and Calories: Effects of Saccharin and Carbohydrates on Hunger and Food Intake in Human Subjects," *Physiology and Behavior* 45 (1989): 1093–99.

19. Erin I. Kleifield and Michael R. Lowe, "Weight Loss and Sweetness Preferences: The Effects of Recent versus Past Weight Loss," *Physiology and Behavior* 49 (1991): 1041.

20. Israel Ramirez, "Rats Discriminate between Starch and Other Substances Having a Similar Texture," *Physiology and Behavior* 53 (1993): 377.

21. Hajime Nagase et al., "Hepatic Glucose-Sensitive Unit Regulation of Glucose-Induced Insulin Secretion in Rats," *Physiology and Behavior* 53 (1993): 142.

22. Judith J. Wurtman et al., "Carbohydrate Craving in Obese People: Suppression by Treatments Affecting Serotoninergic Transmission," *International Journal of Eating Disorders* 1 (1985): 2–15.

23. Ibid., 13.

24. Ibid., 14.

25. Goodrick and Foreyt, "Business of Weight Loss," 1246.

26. Ibid.

27. Homola, *Secrets of Naturally Youthful Health,* 78.

28. Ibid.

29. Lendon Smith, M.D., *Feed Yourself Right* (New York: McGraw-Hill Book Company, 1983), 78.

30. Ibid., 98.

31. Robert Lefever, M.D., and Marie Shafe, "Brain Chemistry: Combinations of Foods in the Blood Trigger Effects Very Similar to Alcohol," *Employee Assistance* 3, no. 8 (March 1991): n.p.

32. Ibid.

33. Larry B. Christensen, *The Food-Mood Connection: Eating Your Way to Happiness* (n.p.: Pro-Health Publications, 1991), 96.

34. Jennifer Cadoff, "Food Cravings," *Glamour,* July 1993, 185.

35. Ibid.

36. Ibid.

37. Ibid.

38. University of California, Berkeley, *The Wellness Encyclopedia* (Boston: Houghton Mifflin Company, 1991), 132.

Chapter 3: What about the Pills?

1. Susan Pack, "Popular Diet Drug Isn't Fine for Everyone, Experts Say," *The News-Times,* 2 December 1996. Available online: http://www.newstimes.com

2. Michael D. Lemonick, "The Mood Molecule," *Time,* 29 September 1997, 80–82.

3. David Stipp, "New Weapons in the War on Fat," *Fortune,* 5 February 1996. Available online: http://www.pathfinder.com/fortune

4. Christine Gorman, "Desperately Seeking a Flab-Fighting Formula," *Time,* 16 January 1995. Available online: http://www.pathfinder.com/time

5. Carolyn O'Neil, "Life after Fen-Phen: Weight-Loss Battle Continues as Before," 21 December 1996. Available online: http://www.cnn.com

6. Stipp, "New Weapons in the War on Fat."

7. Ibid.

8. *Johns Hopkins Family Health Book* (New York: HarperCollins, 1989), 19.

Chapter 4: Just How Dangerous Are Diet Pills?

1. Michael D. Lemonick, "The New Miracle Drug?" *Time,* 23 September 1996. Available online: http://www.pathfinder.com/time

2. Ibid.

3. Robert Langreth and Laura Johannes, "Redux Only for 'Morbidly Obese,' but Marketing Is Lively," *The San Diego Union-Tribune,* 23 November 1996, A31.

4. Susan Pack, "Popular Diet Drug Isn't for Everyone, Experts Say," *The News-Times,* 2 December 1996. Available online: http://www.newstimes.com

5. Eric Adler, "Fen/Phen Skinny Pills Are a Phenomenon," *Fort Worth Star-Telegram,* 23 April 1996. Available online: http://www.startext. net

6. Mary Peterson Kauffold, "Fat Chance: New Anti-obesity Pill Looks Promising but Medicare Experts Hoist a Red Flag," *Chicago Tribune,* 14 July 1996. Available online: http://www.chicagotribune.com

7. Ibid.

8. Ibid.

9. Andrew Bowser, "Obesity Drugs Overprescribed," *The New York Times,* 8 October 1996. Available online: http://www.nytimes.com

10. E-mail posting to author, regarding Fen/Phen. From Joanne P. Ikeda, M. A., R. D., at the Department of Nutritional Sciences, University of California, Berkeley, 14 October 1996.

11. Interneuron Pharmaceuticals, Inc., and Wyeth-Ayerst, *Dexfenfluramine Labeling to Be Updated,* news release, 22 August 1996.

12. Arthur J. Rothafel and Associates, summary of "More Bad News about Fen-Phen Diets," by Elizabeth Cohen, released 1996.

13. E-mail posting to author, regarding Fen/Phen. From Joanne P. Ikeda, M. A., R. D., at the Department of Nutritional Sciences, University of California, Berkeley, 14 October 1996.

14. Arthur J. Rothafel and Associates, summary of "More Bad News."

15. Pack, "Popular Diet Drug."

16. Ibid.

17. Langreth and Johannes, "Redux Only for 'Morbidly Obese,'" A31.

18. Michael D. Lemonick, "The Mood Molecule," *Time,* 29 September 1997, 80.

19. Sandra G. Boodman, "Dieters' Dilemma: What's Left after Withdrawal of Fen/Phen and Redux," *Connecticut Post,* 25 September 1997, B3–B4.

20. Ibid.

21. Ibid.

Chapter 6: Who's Addicted to Food?

1. Nancy Appleton, *Lick the Sugar Habit* (Garden City Park, N.Y.: Avery Publishing Group, 1988), 68.

2. Ibid., 67–68.

3. Andrew Weil, M.D., and Winifred Rosen, *Chocolate to Morphine: Understanding Mind-Active Drugs* (Boston: Houghton Mifflin Company, 1983), 9.

4. Ibid.

5. Ibid.

6. Ibid.

7. Appleton, *Lick the Sugar Habit,* 42–43.

8. Ibid.

9. Ibid.

10. Zoe S. Warwick et al., "Taste and Smell Sensations Enhance the Satiating Effect of Both a High-Carbohydrate and a High-Fat Meal in Humans," *Physiology and Behavior* 53 (1993): 561–62.

11. Jennifer Cadoff, "Food Cravings," *Glamour,* July 1993, 185.

12. Anne Katherine, *Anatomy of a Food Addiction: The Brain Chemistry of Overeating* (New York: Fireside/Parkside, 1991), 36–37.

13. Robert Lefever, M.D., and Marie Shafe, "Brain Chemistry: Combinations of Foods in the Blood Trigger Effects Very Similar to Alcohol," *Employee Assistance* 3, no. 8 (March 1991), n.p.

Chapter 7: I'm Not Like Those People

1. "Meet Gertie Bucket . . . She's One of Europe's Top Models!" *The Sun,* 4 February 1992, 7.

2. Kenneth Silverman et al., "Withdrawal Syndrome after the Double-Blind Cessation of Caffeine Consumption," *The New England Journal of Medicine* 327 (1992): 1109.

3. Ibid.

4. Ibid.

Chapter 9: Finding Your Trigger Foods

1. University of California, Berkeley, *The Wellness Encyclopedia* (Boston: Houghton Mifflin Company, 1991), 131.

2. Ibid.

Index

About the Authors

A recovering food addict, Debbie Danowski has maintained a 150-pound weight loss for over ten years. As an alumnus of a food-addiction treatment center, Danowski has consistently used the recovery program outlined in this book to enjoy the benefits offered by starvation methods and diet pills, without the dangerous health risks. Professionally, Danowski has written more than one hundred articles for national and local publications, including *First for Women, Woman's Day,* and *Seventeen.* She has also spoken about food addiction at countless meetings, seminars, and conferences, including Food Addiction 2000, the first national conference held on the disease. In addition, Danowski was employed by the food-addiction unit of Glenbeigh Hospital of Tampa, a national treatment center, to educate mental health professionals about food addiction recovery. Currently, Danowski is an instructor of media studies at Sacred Heart University in Fairfield, Connecticut, and a member of the university's eating disorders prevention team. Danowski is also a Ph.D. candidate at Capella University in Minneapolis, Minnesota, where she is studying food consumption in film. Danowski has a master's degree from Syracuse University in public communications with an emphasis in television, radio, and film.

A leading expert in the food-addiction field, Pedro Lazaro, M.D., is the former medical director of three addictions hospitals. Prior to that, Dr. Lazaro spent four years as medical director of both the food addiction unit and the entire addictions program at Glenbeigh Hospital of Tampa. Board certified by the American Board of Addictions Medicine and the American Board of Clinical Psychiatry, Dr. Lazaro has over fourteen years experience in the addictions field and has served under Dr. C. Everett Koop as lieutenant commander in the Public Health Service. He currently maintains a general psychiatric practice with two offices in Tampa.